OCN® Certification
Practice Q&A

OCN® Certification
Practice Q&A

SPRINGER PUBLISHING

Springer Publishing Company, LLC
11 West 42nd Street, New York, NY 10036
www.springerpub.com

Acquisitions Editor: Elizabeth Nieginski
Compositor: diacriTech

ISBN: 9780826179081
ebook ISBN: 9780826179098
DOI: 10.1891/9780826179098

22 23 24 25 / 5 4 3 2 1

The author and the publisher of this Work have made every effort to use sources believed to be reliable to provide information that is accurate and compatible with the standards generally accepted at the time of publication. The author and publisher shall not be liable for any special, consequential, or exemplary damages resulting, in whole or in part, from the readers' use of, or reliance on, the information contained in this book. The publisher has no responsibility for the persistence or accuracy of URLs for external or third-party Internet websites referred to in this publication and does not guarantee that any content on such websites is, or will remain, accurate or appropriate.

Contact sales@springerpub.com to receive discount rates on bulk purchases.

Publisher's Note: **New and used products purchased from third-party sellers are not guaranteed for quality, authenticity, or access to any included digital components.**

Printed in the United States of America by Hatteras, Inc.

Contents

Preface

Welcome to *OCN® Certification Practice Q&A*! Congratulations on taking this important step on your journey to becoming a certified oncology nurse. This resource is based on the most recent Oncology Certified Nurse (OCN®) exam blueprint and was developed by experienced oncology nurses. It is designed to help you sharpen your specialty knowledge with 165 practice questions organized by exam subject area, as well as strengthen your knowledge-application and test-taking skills with a 165-question practice exam. It also includes essential information about the OCN® exam, including eligibility requirements, exam subject areas and question distribution, and tips for successful exam preparation.

▶ PART I: PRACTICE QUESTIONS

Part I includes six chapters based on the exam blueprint: Care Continuum, Oncology Nursing Practice, Treatment Modalities, Symptom Management and Palliative Care, Oncologic Emergencies, and Psychosocial Dimensions of Care. Each chapter includes high-quality, exam-style questions and comprehensive answers with rationales that address both correct and incorrect answers. Part I is designed to strengthen your specialty knowledge and is formatted for ultimate studying convenience—answer the questions on each page and simply turn the page for the corresponding answers and rationales. No need to refer to the back of the book for the answers.

▶ PART II: PRACTICE EXAM

Part II includes a 165-question practice exam that aligns with the content domains and question distribution on the most recent OCN® exam blueprint. This practice exam is designed to help you strengthen your knowledge-application and test-taking skills. Maximize your preparation and simulate the exam experience by setting aside 3 hours to complete the practice exam. Comprehensive answers and rationales that address both correct and incorrect answers are located in the chapter immediately following the practice exam.

We know life is busy, and being able to prepare for your exam efficiently and effectively is paramount. This resource will give you the tools and confidence you need to succeed. For additional exam preparation resources, including self-paced online courses, online QBanks, comprehensive review texts, and high-yield study guides, visit www.springerpub.com/examprep. Best of luck to you on your certification journey!

Introduction: OCN® Certification Exam and Tips for Preparation

▶ ELIGIBILITY REQUIREMENTS

The Oncology Certified Nurse (OCN®) exam is developed and administered by the Oncology Nursing Certification Corporation (ONCC®). To qualify to take the exam, you must meet the following requirements:

- A current, active, unencumbered license as a RN in the United States, its territories, or Canada at the time of application and examination.
- A minimum of 2 years (24 months) of experience as an RN within the 4 years (48 months) prior to application.
- A minimum of 2,000 hours of adult oncology nursing practice within the 4 years (48 months) prior to application. Nursing practice may be in clinical practice, nursing administration, education, research, or consultation.
- Completed a minimum of 10 contact hours of nursing continuing education in oncology or an academic elective in oncology nursing within the 3 years (36 months) prior to application. The contact hours must have been provided or formally approved by an acceptable accredited provider or approver of continuing nursing education or nursing continuing professional development. A maximum of 5 of the 10 required contact hours in oncology may be continuing medical education in oncology.

Qualified applicants may submit an online application. Successful candidates will receive an Authorization to Test within 2 weeks of applying and must schedule the exam within a 90-day window. The exam fee is $416; the fee for members of the Oncology Nursing Society (ONS) or the Association of Pediatric Hematology/Oncology Nurses (APHON) is $296. Refer to the ONCC® website for complete eligibility requirements, pricing, and certification information: www.oncc.org/certifications/oncology-certified-nurse-ocn.

▶ ABOUT THE EXAMINATION

The OCN® exam takes 3 hours and consists of 165 multiple-choice questions with four answer options. You must select the single best answer. See Table 1 for exam content domains and question distribution. For more detailed exam content information, refer to the OCN® Test Content Outline at www.oncc.org/files/2022OCNOutline.pdf.

Table 1. OCN® Exam Content Domains and Question Distribution

Content Domain	Percentage of Questions
Care Continuum	19%
Oncology Nursing Practice	17%
Treatment Modalities	19%
Symptom Management and Palliative Care	21%
Oncologic Emergencies	12%
Psychosocial Dimensions of Care	12%

▶ TIPS FOR EXAM PREPARATION

You know the old joke about how to get to Carnegie Hall—practice, practice, practice! The same is true when seeking certification. Practice and preparation are key to your success on exam day. Here are 10 tips to help you prepare:

1. Allow at least 6 months to fully prepare for the exam. Do not rely on last-minute cramming sessions.
2. Thoroughly review the OCN® Test Content Outline so that you know exactly what to expect. Pay close attention to the content domains, subdomains, and topics. Identify your strengths, weaknesses, and knowledge gaps, so you know where to focus your studies. Review all of the supplementary resources available on the ONCC® website.
3. Create a study timeline with weekly or monthly study tasks. Be as specific as possible—identify *what* you will study, *how* you will study, and *when* you will study.
4. Use several exam prep resources that provide different benefits. For example, use a comprehensive review to build your specialty knowledge, use this resource and other question banks to strengthen your knowledge-application and test-taking skills, and use a high-yield review to brush up on key concepts in the days leading up to the exam. Springer Publishing offers a wide range of print and online exam prep products to suit all of your study needs; visit www.springerpub.com/examprep.
5. Assess your level of knowledge and performance on practice questions and exams. Carefully consider why you may be missing certain questions. Continually analyze your strengths, weaknesses, and knowledge gaps, and adjust your study plan accordingly.
6. Minimize distraction as much as possible while you are studying. You will feel more calm, centered, and focused, which will lead to increased knowledge retention.
7. Engage in stress-reducing activities, particularly in the month leading up to the exam. Yoga, stretching, and deep-breathing exercises can be beneficial. If you are feeling frustrated or anxious while studying, take a break. Go for a walk, play with your child or pet, or finish a chore that has been weighing on you. Wait until you feel more refreshed before returning to study.

8. Focus on your health in the weeks and days before the exam. Eat balanced meals, stay hydrated, and minimize alcohol consumption. Get as much sleep as possible, particularly the night before the exam.
9. Eat a light meal before the exam but limit your liquid consumption. The clock does not stop for restroom breaks! Ensure that you know exactly where you are going and how long it will take to get there. Leave with plenty of time to spare to reduce travel-related stress and ensure that you arrive on time.
10. Remind yourself to relax and stay calm. You have prepared, and you know your stuff. Visualize the success that is just ahead of you and make it happen. When you pass, celebrate!

Pass Guarantee

If you use this resource to prepare for your exam and you do not pass, you may return it for a refund of your full purchase price. To receive a refund, you must return your product along with a copy of your original receipt and exam score report. Product must be returned and received within 180 days of the original purchase date. This excludes tax, shipping, and handling. One offer per person and address. Refunds will be issued within 8 weeks from acceptance and approval. This offer is valid for U.S. residents only. Void where prohibited. To initiate a refund, please contact customer service at CS@springerpub.com.

Part I
Practice Questions and Answers
With Rationales

Care Continuum

1. Which of the following is an example of a late-onset side effect from cancer treatment?

    A. Nausea
    B. Hair loss
    C. Osteoporosis
    D. Mouth sores

2. The top five most commonly diagnosed cancers worldwide are:

    A. Breast, lung, colorectal, stomach, and prostate
    B. Breast, lung, colorectal, uterine, and prostate
    C. Breast, melanoma, lung, stomach, and prostate
    D. Breast, cervical, lung, melanoma, and prostate

3. Cancer is a leading cause of death in the United States, second only to:

    A. Diabetes
    B. Heart disease
    C. Injuries and accidents
    D. Respiratory disease

4. The 5-year survival rate is highest for which types of cancer in the United States?

    A. Liver, lung, and pancreatic cancers
    B. Liver and breast cancers and chronic myeloid leukemia
    C. Prostate and breast cancers and melanoma
    D. Lung and breast cancers and melanoma

5. The single most preventable cause of disease and premature death in the United States is:

    A. Obesity
    B. Tobacco use
    C. Alcohol consumption
    D. UV radiation exposure

1. C) Osteoporosis
Late-onset side effects are symptoms that develop later in a patient's cancer journey, usually after treatment has ended. Exposure to chemotherapy and radiation can result in bone loss and increases the risk of osteoporosis. Nausea, hair loss, and mouth sores are examples of acute side effects that can occur during cancer treatment. They typically subside as treatment ends.

2. A) Breast, lung, colorectal, stomach, and prostate
The top five most commonly diagnosed cancers worldwide are breast, lung, colorectal, stomach, and prostate, making up nearly half of all cases diagnosed. The top five most commonly diagnosed cancers in the United States are breast, prostate, lung, colorectal, and uterine. Although melanoma is not one of the most common cancers, its incidence is increasing. Cervical cancer is not one of the most commonly diagnosed cancers, but it is the second leading cause of death in women ages 20 to 39 years.

3. B) Heart disease
Cancer is a leading cause of death, second only to heart disease. According to the Centers for Disease Control and Prevention, the third most common cause of death is accidents and unintentional injuries. The fourth most common cause of death is respiratory diseases.

4. C) Prostate and breast cancers and melanoma
The 5-year survival rate is highest for prostate cancer, melanoma, and female breast cancer. Survival is lowest for liver, lung, and pancreatic cancers. The survival rate for chronic myeloid leukemia has increased significantly as well, but it is not considered to have one of the highest survival rates.

5. B) Tobacco use
Tobacco use, including smoking, exposure to secondhand smoke, and use of smokeless tobacco, is the largest preventable cause of disease and premature death in the United States. Smoking increases the risk of cancer of the lungs, mouth, nasal and oral cavities, larynx, pharynx, esophagus, stomach, colorectum, liver, pancreas, kidneys, bladder, uterus, cervix, and ovaries, as well as the risk of acute myeloid leukemia. Obesity, alcohol consumption, and UV exposure are all examples of cancer risk factors, but tobacco use is the largest preventable cause.

6. The leading cause of oral cancers is:

   A. Smoking
   B. Alcohol consumption
   C. Human papillomavirus (HPV)-16
   D. *Helicobacter pylori*

7. Which of the following is a modifiable risk factor in the prevention of cancer?

   A. Asbestos exposure
   B. Radiation exposure
   C. Genetics
   D. Virus exposure

8. "I do not think that I need to reduce my alcohol intake to lower my chances of getting cancer." This statement from a patient is an example of which component of the health belief model?

   A. Perceived barriers to preventive action
   B. Perceived benefits of preventive behavior
   C. Perceived severity of cancer
   D. Perceived susceptibility to cancer

9. Human papillomavirus (HPV) vaccination is an example of which type of cancer prevention?

   A. Primary prevention
   B. Tertiary prevention
   C. Primordial prevention
   D. Secondary prevention

(See answers next page.)

6. C) Human papillomavirus (HPV)-16

HPV-16, a type of human papillomavirus, is the leading cause of oral cancers. It is found substantially in squamous cell carcinomas of the soft palate, tonsils, and base of the tongue. Alcohol consumption and smoking are also risk factors in the development of oral cancer but are not the leading causes. *Helicobacter pylori* is associated with cancer of the stomach.

7. D) Virus exposure

Modifiable risk factors are those that can be changed or avoided. Virus exposure is considered a modifiable risk factor as there are multiple vaccines available to aid in protection against infection. For example, the hepatitis B virus is associated with cirrhosis and liver cancer. The hepatitis B vaccination is a primary prevention strategy. Nonmodifiable risk factors are those that cannot be changed. Asbestos exposure is considered a nonmodifiable risk factor and is associated with occupational exposures; occupations include mining, construction, and firefighting, as well as work associated with railroads, shipyards, boiler plants, refineries, and paper, textile, and steel mills. Genetics and radiation exposure, such as to radon gas and x-rays, are also considered nonmodifiable risk factors.

8. B) Perceived benefits of preventive behavior

The health belief model is useful to assess patients for motivation for preventive behavior. Perceived benefits of preventive behavior include asking the patient if they think they can decrease their risk of developing cancer by modifying certain risk factors. This patient does not feel that reducing alcohol intake would decrease their risk. Perceived barriers to action include identifying problems that would prevent the patient from reducing risk factors, such as addiction to alcohol and being unable to reduce intake. Perceived severity of cancer addresses how serious the patient feels cancer is and their willingness to modify risk behavior. Perceived susceptibility to cancer assesses how likely a patient feels they are to develop cancer. An example would be the patient saying, "That will never happen to me."

9. A) Primary prevention

Primary prevention reduces risk factors or increases an individual's resistance to them. Vaccinations are used to limit the incidence of cancer development by protecting from infection. Primordial prevention refers to avoiding the development of risk factors in the first place (e.g., abstaining from sexual behavior to avoid virus infection). Secondary prevention refers to early detection and treatment of cancer through screening in asymptomatic individuals. Tertiary prevention includes therapy to improve outcomes and decrease mortality in affected individuals.

10. A 30-year-old patient with no personal history of breast cancer but whose mother was diagnosed with breast cancer and is positive for the *BRCA1* gene mutation would be advised to:

    A. Begin mammography annually at age 35 years

    B. Begin annual mammography now

    C. Begin mammography now and continue every other year

    D. Begin annual mammography with MRI now

11. A patient is discussing early cancer screening with colonoscopy for colorectal cancer (CRC). The patient's father is 59 years old and has recently been diagnosed with CRC. The appropriate recommendation by the nurse would be colonoscopy every:

    A. 10 years beginning at age 40 years

    B. 5 years beginning at age 40 years

    C. 5 years beginning at age 45 years

    D. 10 years beginning at age 45 years

12. A 19-year-old sexually active patient is scheduled for a physical examination. Which of the following is correct regarding cervical cancer screening for this patient?

    A. Consider human papillomavirus (HPV) testing

    B. Initiate Pap testing

    C. Perform no screening

    D. Initiate screening with HPV and Pap tests

13. Which of the following is considered a modifiable risk factor for the prevention of colon cancer?

    A. Exposure to secondhand smoke

    B. Sex

    C. Age

    D. Vegetable consumption

(See answers next page.)

10. D) Begin annual mammography with MRI now

A patient with a *BRCA1* or *BRCA2* gene mutation as well as a first-degree relative with cancer is considered high risk. Screening recommendations include annual mammography and MRI starting at age 30 years. Average-risk patients are defined as those with no genetic mutations or personal or strong family history of breast cancer. These women are given the option to start screening with mammography every year beginning at age 40 years. Women age 55 years and older at average risk are given the option to switch to mammography screening every other year or to continue with yearly mammograms.

11. B) 5 years beginning at age 40 years

A patient with a history of colorectal cancer in any first-degree relative before age 60 years, or in at least two second-degree relatives at any age, should begin colonoscopy every 5 years at age of 40 years, or 10 years before the youngest diagnosis, whichever comes first. Average-risk populations are defined as having no personal or family history and no history of inflammatory bowel disease. Recommendations for average-risk populations are to begin regular screening with colonoscopy every 10 years beginning at age 45 years.

12. C) Perform no screening

Screening is not recommended for patients younger than 21 years, regardless of sexual history. Beginning at age 21 years, recommendations are to perform Pap tests every 3 years. Yearly screening is no longer recommended because it generally takes 10 to 20 years for cervical cancer to develop. HPV testing is only needed after an abnormal Pap result.

13. D) Vegetable consumption

Choosing a diet rich in vegetables, as well as whole fruit and other high-fiber foods, decreases the risk of developing colon cancer. Exposure to secondhand smoke is a modifiable risk factor for the prevention of lung cancer and cardiovascular disease. Sex and age are examples of nonmodifiable risk factors.

14. The preferred screening method for colorectal cancer is:

  A. Stool DNA test
  B. Colonoscopy
  C. Barium enema
  D. CT colonography

15. At which point is a patient considered a cancer survivor?

  A. From the time of diagnosis through the rest of their life
  B. After their last treatment and through the rest of their life
  C. After their last test results and exams show no evidence of disease
  D. After they feel they have completed their cancer care journey

16. Which statement is true regarding fear of recurrence in cancer survivors?

  A. It occurs more commonly in older survivors
  B. It leads to better adherence to follow-up care
  C. It is associated with improved daily functioning
  D. It can negatively impact quality of life

17. Surveillance recommendations for patients who have received chest radiation as a child, adolescent, or young adult include:

  A. Mammogram and MRI yearly, beginning 8 years after radiation or at age 25 years, whichever occurs last
  B. Mammogram and MRI every other year, beginning 8 years after radiation or at age 25 years, whichever occurs last
  C. Mammogram yearly with MRI every other year, beginning 8 years after radiation or at age 25 years, whichever occurs first
  D. Mammogram and MRI yearly, beginning 8 years after radiation or at age 25 years, whichever occurs first

(See answers next page.)

14. B) Colonoscopy

Colonoscopy is the preferred method for colorectal cancer screening because it allows for a more thorough examination of the large intestine and the rectum, visualizing most lesions and polyps. Because of this, colonoscopy recommendation for the average-risk population is every 10 years. Stool DNA tests assess for mutations shed in stool that are associated with lesions. These tests are not widely available and require more frequent testing (every 3 years). Barium enemas are noninvasive; however, they do not allow for biopsy or removal of lesions and are required every 5 years. CT colonography is a good option for older adults and frail patients, however, there are insufficient data to support it as a solitary screening method at this time. It also is recommended more frequently (every 5 years). With stool DNA tests, barium enemas, and CT colonography, any positive test would require a colonoscopy.

15. A) From the time of diagnosis through the rest of their life

A patient is considered a cancer survivor from the time of diagnosis through the rest of their life, regardless of treatments, test results, and exams.

16. D) It can negatively impact quality of life

The fear of recurrence can negatively impact a cancer survivor's quality of life. It can lead to poor adherence to follow-up recommendations and is associated with depression and impaired daily functioning. Fear of recurrence more often occurs in younger survivors.

17. A) Mammogram and MRI yearly, beginning 8 years after radiation or at age 25 years, whichever occurs last

Patients who received chest radiation as a child or young adult are at risk of developing breast cancer. Current guidelines recommend yearly MRI with mammogram beginning 8 years after radiation or at age 25, whichever occurs last. Additional screening includes monthly breast self-exams beginning at puberty and yearly clinical breast exams beginning at age 25 years.

18. While a patient's chemotherapy toxicity symptoms are being assessed, the patient states that they are having difficulty grasping objects and buttoning their clothes. They complain of constant hand, wrist, and foot pain. Which action demonstrates the nurse's awareness of long-term effects from cancer treatment?

    A. Instruct patient to soak hands and feet in warm water daily and regularly apply a fragrance-free lotion
    B. Refer the patient to physical therapy to allow for continued treatment
    C. Withhold treatment and notify the provider, anticipating changes in dosing
    D. Remind the patient that neuropathy is a common side effect of cancer treatment, often subsiding once treatment has ended

19. A patient presents with fatigue, pallor, and petechiae to lower extremities. They report having received cyclophosphamide treatment as a young adult. The nurse anticipates which of the following?

    A. Bone marrow exam
    B. Brain MRI
    C. Ultrasound to spleen
    D. Lumbar puncture

20. A nurse is providing education to a patient with oropharyngeal cancer. Which late effect must the patient be aware of to prevent an increase in dental caries, halitosis, and changes in voice and taste?

    A. Trismus
    B. Xerostomia
    C. Osteoradionecrosis of the jaw
    D. Dysphagia

21. A nurse assessing a patient for signs of impending death would expect to find:

    A. Increased urine output
    B. Hyper-responsiveness to visual stimuli
    C. Reactive pupils
    D. Cheyne–Stokes respiration

(See answers next page.)

18. C) Withhold treatment and notify the provider, anticipating changes in dosing

The patient is experiencing symptoms of chemotherapy-induced peripheral neuropathy (CIPN). To prevent long-term effects such as motor function impairment, balance issues, and chronic pain, the nurse must report these symptoms and anticipate dose modification, withholding, or discontinuation of the causative agent. Physical therapy or soaking in warm water may help with symptoms; however, the primary goal is to prevent long-term damage from occurring. It is true that with the completion of some therapies, CIPN improves or resolves; however, there must be an assessment by the provider to determine if continuation is safe.

19. A) Bone marrow exam

Based on the patient's history and current physical symptoms, the nurse should suspect that development of myelodysplasia or acute myeloid leukemia has occurred as a late effect of cyclophosphamide treatment. Appropriate action would be a bone marrow exam along with a complete blood count to assess bone marrow function. Petechiae, easy bruising, pallor, and fatigue are common signs of low platelets and red blood cells.

20. B) Xerostomia

Oropharyngeal cancer patients can experience many later-term effects from cancer treatment and radiation. Xerostomia occurs when there is damage to the salivary glands. It is described as dry mouth, thick saliva, burning pain, mouth sores, difficulty chewing, halitosis, increased infections and dental caries, and changes in voice and taste. Educate patients about saliva stimulants, proper dental hygiene, decreasing alcohol and caffeine intake, and tobacco cessation. Trismus occurs as a result of damage to the mastication muscles and may limit range of motion in a patient's jaws, leading to difficulty speaking, chewing, and swallowing. Educate patients about range-of-motion exercises, effective pain management, and use of tongue blades and mouth-opening devices. Osteoradionecrosis of the jaw can occur from the bones not healing after radiation. Remind the patient about dental assessments and proper dental hygiene, proper nutrition, and managing their comorbidities. Dysphagia, or difficulty swallowing, can occur from surgery or radiation. Physical therapy can offer support and healing.

21. D) Cheyne–Stokes respiration

Cheyne–Stokes respiration is a type of breathing characterized by cyclical episodes of apnea and hyperventilation and is a clinical sign of impending death. Other signs of impending death include decreased urine output, decreased response to visual stimuli, increased terminal secretions, and nonreactive pupils. Nurses can also expect pulselessness to radial artery and terminal secretions. Having awareness of impending death allows the nurse to educate and support the patient's family and loved ones through the dying process.

22. A nurse is reviewing a survivorship care plan for a patient with melanoma who completed immunotherapy treatment. The patient had a delay during treatment and was treated with corticosteroids for pneumonitis. The nurse would ensure that which of the following is performed?

    A. Echocardiogram
    B. Dual-energy x-ray absorptiometry (DEXA) scan
    C. Chest x-ray
    D. Hemoglobin A1C

23. At which time should an advance directive be completed?

    A. At the time of receiving a terminal diagnosis
    B. Upon a hospital admission for any cause
    C. When a person is considered healthy
    D. Once comfort care is initiated

24. A nurse is discussing hospice care with a patient's spouse. Which statement made by the spouse alerts the nurse that more education is needed?

    A. "We have Medicare, so I am not worried about how we will afford hospice care."
    B. "We want to start hospice care and stop chemotherapy treatments."
    C. "Physical therapy has helped with pain management, and we don't want to lose that."
    D. "We understand that it requires a prognosis of 6 months or less to live, but that can be extended if needed."

25. A patient with extensive lung cancer is experiencing refractory pain despite multiple interventions. The patient has become angry and distressed toward their care providers. They have started missing appointments, and their care has become compromised as a result. Which of the following nursing interventions would best support the patient at this time?

    A. Consult an anger management professional for de-escalation support
    B. Initiate the involvement of an interdisciplinary team
    C. Initiate a referral to the pain management clinic
    D. Request a consult for palliative care services

(See answers next page.)

22. B) Dual-energy x-ray absorptiometry (DEXA) scan

Management of immune-related adverse events may require the use of systemic corticosteroids. Corticosteroid use is associated with long-term effects, such as the development of osteoporosis. Patients that received corticosteroids should have DEXA scan monitoring as part of their care plans to monitor for the development of osteoporosis. Echocardiograms, chest x-rays, and hemoglobin A1C monitoring are not routinely ordered as survivorship care for patients receiving immunotherapy.

23. C) When a person is considered healthy

An advance directive is a legal document that explains how a person wants medical decisions to be made in the event that they cannot make them for themselves. It is meant to help people plan ahead and guide their loved ones in making decisions about the care they desire. Advance directives are most advantageous when filled out during a healthy state, before the person becomes too ill or injured to make medical decisions.

24. C) "Physical therapy has helped with pain management, and we don't want to lose that."

Medicare covers hospice care as long as the patient meets the eligibility requirements. The criteria for hospice eligibility includes a prognosis of 6 months or less to live, and the agreement that the terminal illness will no longer be treated for cure (chemotherapy), but that the whole body will be treated to improve quality of life. Physical therapy is included as a hospice service, as it aids in pain management and improvement of quality of life. After 6 months, hospice care can continue as long as the hospice doctor recertifies that the patient remains terminally ill.

25. B) Initiate the involvement of an interdisciplinary team

An interdisciplinary team is comprised of physicians, nurses, social workers, spiritual care providers, dieticians, and other healthcare professionals who come together to identify and set goals to meet the needs of patients and their caregivers. This would be the most beneficial intervention because the patient will receive the expertise of multiple professions, allowing for all options to be discussed. Pain clinic and palliative care services would be included in this process. De-escalation training is useful for care providers but would not be the most helpful intervention for the patient at this point in their care. Focus should be on supporting the patient's underlying issues (e.g., better pain management, which would lead to less anger and better adherence to care).

26. A patient who has been battling leukemia is admitted to the hospital with sepsis and a poor prognosis. The patient and family decide that they would prefer to stay on the oncology unit rather than go to the ICU. The patient is not expected to survive the night. What is the nurse's most appropriate action?

    A. Encourage the family to leave the room to allow the patient to rest peacefully as much as possible
    B. Help the family gather the patient's personal belongings in preparation for death
    C. Leave the family alone to spend time with their loved one
    D. Ask the family what their needs are, and provide information on the dying process

27. Which types of cancer have the lowest survival rate in the United States?

    A. Liver, lung, and pancreatic cancers
    B. Lung and breast cancers and melanoma
    C. Prostate and breast cancers and melanoma
    D. Liver and breast cancers and chronic myeloid leukemia

28. "I am having trouble reducing my alcohol intake because of my addiction." This statement from a patient is an example of which component of the health belief model?

    A. Perceived barriers to preventive action
    B. Perceived benefits of preventive behavior
    C. Perceived severity of cancer
    D. Perceived susceptibility to cancer

29. A patient receiving an aromatase inhibitor has an increased risk of developing which late effect?

    A. Alopecia
    B. Peripheral neuropathy
    C. Osteoporosis
    D. Constipation

(See answers next page.)

26. D) Ask the family what their needs are, and provide information on the dying process

Families of dying patients often need support in understanding what to expect during the dying process. Asking them their needs will allow the family to feel supported, and encouraging them to stay with the patient during the dying process will help later with their grief. Asking them their needs will also help the nurse to determine how much they would like to be alone with their loved one, as every family is different. It is also a good idea to talk about what postmortem care will look like and to what extent the families would like to be involved. Offering to help gather patient's belongings should be done after death.

27. A) Liver, lung, and pancreatic cancers

Cancers with the lowest survival rate in the United States are liver, lung, and pancreatic cancers. Cancers with the highest survival rate are prostate cancer, melanoma, and female breast cancer. The survival rate for chronic myeloid leukemia has increased significantly and so is not considered one of the lowest.

28. A) Perceived barriers to preventive action

The health belief model is useful to assess patients for motivation for preventive behavior. Perceived barriers to action include identifying problems that would prevent the patient from reducing risk factors, such as addiction to alcohol and being unable to reduce intake. Perceived benefits of preventive behavior include asking the patient if they think they can decrease their risk of developing cancer by modifying certain risk factors. Perceived severity of cancer addresses how serious the patient feels cancer is and their willingness to modify risk behavior. Perceived susceptibility to cancer assesses how likely a patient believes they are to develop cancer.

29. C) Osteoporosis

Aromatase inhibitor use decreases bone mineral density over time, increasing a patient's risk for osteoporosis. Alopecia, peripheral neuropathy, and constipation are not typical side effects of aromatase inhibitors.

30. A nurse is providing education to a patient with oropharyngeal cancer. Which late effect is the nurse addressing when educating about the importance of range-of-motion exercises throughout and beyond completion of treatment?

A. Trismus

B. Xerostomia

C. Osteoradionecrosis of the jaw

D. Dysphagia

(See answers next page.)

30. A) Trismus

Oropharyngeal cancer patients can experience many later-term effects from cancer treatment and radiation. Trismus occurs as a result of damage to the mastication muscles and may limit range of motion in patient's jaws, leading to difficulty speaking, chewing, or swallowing. Patients should be educated about range-of-motion exercises, effective pain management, and the use of tongue blades and mouth-opening devices. Xerostomia occurs when there is damage to the salivary glands. It is described as dry mouth, thick saliva, burning pain, mouth sores, difficulty chewing, halitosis, increased infections and dental caries, and changes in voice and taste. Educate patients about saliva stimulants, proper dental hygiene, decreasing alcohol and caffeine intake, and tobacco cessation. Osteoradionecrosis of the jaw can occur from the bones not healing after radiation. Remind the patient about dental assessments and proper dental hygiene, proper nutrition, and managing comorbidities. Dysphagia, or difficulty swallowing, can occur from surgery or radiation. Physical therapy can offer support and healing.

Oncology Nursing Practice

2

1. The Philadelphia chromosome is an example of a:

    A. Proto-oncogene
    B. Translocation
    C. Tumor suppressor gene
    D. Caretaker gene

2. A large amount of telomerase is believed to contribute to what feature of cancer cells?

    A. Extended survival
    B. Cell mutation
    C. Chromosome translocation
    D. Angiogenesis

3. What is considered part of the primary lymphoid system?

    A. Tonsils
    B. Thymus
    C. Spleen
    D. Thyroid

4. Innate immunity differs from adaptive immunity in that innate immunity:

    A. Does not cause an inflammatory response
    B. Differentiates between pathogens
    C. Does not require previous exposure to activate
    D. Occurs later in the immune cascade

5. Postprocedure education for a patient undergoing a breast biopsy includes:

    A. Not lifting anything heavier than 5 pounds for the first 3 days
    B. Bathing, swimming, and soaking as typically done before the procedure
    C. Applying a heating pad several times a day to help with bruising and swelling
    D. Removing the bandage and steristrips before showering

1. B) Translocation
The Philadelphia chromosome, which occurs in chronic myeloid leukemia, is an example of a chromosome translocation in which part of one chromosome switches to another chromosome during cell division. A proto-oncogene is a gene that controls the normal growth of cells. A tumor suppressor gene prevents uncontrolled cell proliferation. A caretaker gene repairs defects in DNA.

2. A) Extended survival
Telomerase is the enzyme responsible for adding telomeres, or protective DNA, to the ends of chromosomes. The high levels of telomerase in cancer cells increase the number of telomere segments, allowing the cells to live longer and continue to replicate. Telomerase does not directly contribute to cell mutation, chromosome translocation, or angiogenesis.

3. B) Thymus
The primary lymphoid system enables the maturation of lymphocytes. The thymus, a primary lymphoid organ, is involved in the maturation of T-cells. The spleen, which responds to antigens in the blood, is a secondary lymphoid organ. The tonsils and thyroid gland are not considered part of the lymphoid organs or tissues.

4. C) Does not require previous exposure to activate
Innate immunity, also known as natural immunity, does not require previous exposure to a foreign substance in order to become activated, while adaptive immunity does. The inflammatory response is a component of innate immunity but not adaptive immunity. Unlike adaptive immunity, innate immunity does not differentiate between pathogens. Innate immunity is the initial line of immune defense, while adaptive immunity occurs in the later stages of the immune response.

5. A) Not lifting anything heavier than 5 pounds for the first 3 days
Care recommendations after a breast biopsy include not lifting anything heavier than 5 pounds for the first 3 days. They also include avoiding strenuous activity like running. Bathing, swimming, or soaking for the first few days should be avoided as well, to prevent infection at the biopsy site. It is permitted to shower after 24 hours, letting the water run over the biopsy site and then patting dry. Prior to showering, the patient should remove the bandage but leave the steristrips in place to fall off on their own. If after 3 days the steristrips have not fallen off, they may be removed at that time. It is common in the first 24 to 48 hours for swelling and bruising to occur. Recommendations include icing the area for 10 to 15 minutes several times in that initial period.

6. Which of the following classifications of breast cancer is considered nonmalignant?

   A. Ductal carcinoma in situ (DCIS)
   B. Invasive ductal carcinoma
   C. Inflammatory breast cancer
   D. Lobular carcinoma

7. A nurse is discussing hormone replacement therapy with a patient with breast cancer. Which of the following statements by the patient alerts the nurse that more education is needed?

   A. "Hormone replacement therapy depends on my menopause status."
   B. "I might be taking tamoxifen and anastrozole concurrently."
   C. "Hormone therapy will decrease my estrogen and progesterone levels."
   D. "I take sertraline, which may affect the way tamoxifen works."

8. Which type of clinical trial aims to improve ways of detecting disease earlier in healthy people?

   A. Prevention
   B. Diagnostic
   C. Treatment
   D. Screening

9. Which of the following statements is inaccurate regarding participation in clinical trials?

   A. Patients choose to participate due to lack of available treatment options
   B. Clinical trials allow access to treatment that patients would otherwise be unable to afford
   C. Patients may be entered in certain clinical trials without their knowing
   D. Patients join with hope they will be given better treatment than the current standard

(See answers next page.)

6. A) Ductal carcinoma in situ (DCIS)

DCIS is considered a nonmalignant breast cancer because it is manageable and treatable. DCIS can become invasive if not removed; therefore, surgery is recommended. Invasive ductal carcinoma is the most common type of breast cancer; prognosis is variable, depending on cellular characteristics. Inflammatory breast cancer is an aggressive subtype and manifests with edema in the skin and dermal lymphatic invasion of the breast, which mimics mastitis. Lobular carcinoma has a prognosis similar to invasive ductal carcinoma and is capable of metastasis to unusual surfaces, such as the pericardium, ovary, abdomen, uterus, eye, and stomach.

7. B) "I might be taking tamoxifen and anastrozole concurrently."

Tamoxifen and aromatase inhibitors (AIs), such as anastrozole and letrozole, are not given concurrently. The type of hormone replacement therapy depends on a patient's menopausal status at diagnosis. Typically, a premenopausal patient will be prescribed tamoxifen for 5 to 10 years and an AI (not concurrently) if ovarian suppression or ablation occurred. In a postmenopausal patient, an AI and tamoxifen are typically prescribed; however, the order in which they are given is unclear and variable. Some patients start with an AI for 5 years followed by tamoxifen for 5 years, or in reverse order. Hormone therapy will decrease estrogen and progesterone concentrations, or prevent interactions with their receptors, resulting in hot flashes and mood changes. Certain selective serotonin reuptake inhibitors (SSRIs) reduce tamoxifen efficacy. The preferred SSRIs when taking tamoxifen are citalopram, escitalopram, and venlafaxine. This patient is taking sertraline (Zoloft) and therefore should discuss this with their provider.

8. D) Screening

Clinical trials that focus on screening assess for new and improved ways to detect disease and health conditions earlier in healthy people. Examples include obtaining tissue samples, genetic testing, imaging tests, health histories, and physical examinations. Clinical trials that focus on prevention evaluate the effectiveness of ways to reduce the risk of developing disease or to prevent a disease from returning. Examples are lifestyle changes, medications, and vaccines. Diagnostic clinical trials aim to develop better tests and procedures to identify and diagnose disease. Treatment-focused clinical trials test new treatments or devices, new drug combinations, and new approaches to surgery and radiation treatment. These trials are categorized by phases.

9. C) Patients may be entered in certain clinical trials without their knowing

Patients must voluntarily agree to enter a clinical trial. The informed consent process includes the sharing of information about the nature of the research and the evaluation of the patient's comprehension of that information, as well as their voluntary decision to participate.

10. In which section of a clinical research protocol would a nurse find information about other treatments a patient can or cannot receive while on a clinical trial?

  A. Abstract

  B. Eligibility assessment and enrollment

  C. Study implementation

  D. Supportive care

11. A nurse is reviewing a drug currently in a clinical trial and notes that the study has thousands of participants and is being conducted in multiple locations. It includes a control group and uses randomization. The drug is being compared with the current standard of treatment. The nurse concludes that the drug is in which phase of the clinical trial?

  A. Phase 1

  B. Phase 2

  C. Phase 3

  D. Phase 4

12. Which of the following is true regarding the safe handling of antineoplastic agents?

  A. Oral chemotherapy agents are safer than parenteral chemotherapy agents

  B. It is safe to wear one pair of gloves when administering oral chemotherapy agents

  C. Personal protective equipment (PPE) should be worn when handling patient waste for 24 hours after last chemotherapy dose

  D. Parenteral and oral chemotherapy administration requires the same safe handling

(See answers next page.)

10. C) Study implementation

The study implementation section of a research protocol provides information about the study and treatment plan, such as the study design, how the intervention will be given, specimen collection, reasons a patient might be taken off a study, and other treatments a patient may or may not receive while on the study. The abstract section is a summary of the study background, objectives, eligibility, and design. The eligibility assessment and enrollment section provides further details on inclusion and exclusion criteria for joining a study. The supportive care section provides guidance on managing the patient's symptoms while participating in the study. Other sections of a protocol include title page, table of contents, data collection, protection procedures, and drug information.

11. C) Phase 3

Clinical trials have three main phases, plus a fourth phase that takes place after the drug enters the market. The goal of phase 3 is to compare the new drug with the current standard treatment. Studies include large numbers of people (hundreds to thousands), are conducted in multiple locations, and use randomization to assign patients to control and treatment groups. Phase 1 studies are small—15 to 60 patients who all receive the same study drug. The goal of this phase is to determine a dose or dosing schedule that is safe for humans, called the maximum tolerated dose. In phase 2, the drug effectiveness is evaluated. Studies are larger than in phase 1, usually 100 to 300 patients, and include patients for whom the current standard of care is not effective for their diagnosis. Phase 4 occurs after the drug enters the market and becomes available to the general public. Evaluation of risks, benefits, and uses in real-life scenarios occurs, and this involves thousands of patients.

12. D) Parenteral and oral chemotherapy administration requires the same safe handling

It is a common misconception that oral chemotherapy administration is safer than parenteral chemotherapy administration. Continuous exposure to oral chemotherapy increases the risk of contact dermatitis, spontaneous abortion, liver damage, and respiratory tissue damage. PPE use standards should be the same for both routes of administration. This includes double gloving with chemotherapy-approved gloves, wearing low-permeability gowns, and wearing a face shield if there is a risk of splashing. When handling patient waste, PPE should be worn for at least 48 hours or longer after the last chemotherapy dose.

13. A nurse is preparing to administer a new regimen to a patient who does not speak English and with whom the nurse is unable to communicate clearly. It is late in the day, and the nurse is feeling rushed to start the infusion but is concerned that the patient does not understand the new treatment plan and may be uncomfortable. Rather than hanging the medication, the nurse finds a translator. It takes longer to get the infusion started, but the patient is able to ask questions and express understanding. Which ethical principle drove the nurse's action to delay treatment until the patient was able to ask questions and better understand?

    A. Veracity

    B. Autonomy

    C. Fidelity

    D. Justice

14. Which of the following is true regarding safeguards and strategies to prevent medication errors?

    A. Verbal orders are permitted if they allow more timely medication administration

    B. Standardized preprinted or electronic orders are preferred to handwritten orders

    C. Abbreviations and acronyms are used for easier interpretation of orders

    D. Variance from standard regimens does not pose any risk for medication errors

15. What is the "E" in the ABCDEs of mole and melanoma recognition?

    A. Ever-changing

    B. Evolving

    C. Evergreen

    D. Energized

16. Which of the following is true regarding UV radiation (UVR) and the pathophysiology of skin cancer?

    A. UVR comes solely from sun exposure

    B. UVR causes DNA damage, resulting in mutations of key cancer genes

    C. UVA radiation is absorbed in the epidermis

    D. UVB radiation passes deeper into the skin than UVA

(See answers next page.)

13. A) Veracity

Veracity is providing accurate information and truth telling. Explaining treatment in understandable terms before it is initiated is an example of veracity. The nurse found support to make sure the patient was given accurate information and felt that they had all of the necessary information. Autonomy is independent decision-making by an individual in accordance with their best interest. Respecting an individual's choice, even if it is different from one's own, is an example of autonomy. Fidelity is faithfulness to promises made, such as following up as promised. Justice describes equitable distribution of available resources regardless of ability to pay, culture, or socioeconomic status.

14. B) Standardized preprinted or electronic orders are preferred to handwritten orders

Medication errors cause injury and death daily, and safeguards and strategies must be implemented to prevent them. Using preprinted or electronic order sets has been shown to increase evidence-based oncology care and decrease errors. Verbal orders for chemotherapy, immunotherapy, and targeted therapy are not permitted except to hold or stop drugs. Abbreviations and acronyms lead to ambiguous and unclear orders and should be avoided. Orders should be regimen based and include the elements outlined by current safety standards. Policies should be in place when a provider orders regimens that vary from standard regimens. For example, the prescriber is required to document supporting references for the variance.

15. B) Evolving

The ABCDEs of melanoma is an acronym used for signs and symptoms of melanoma. "E" is for evolving. Normal moles should not change in size, shape, or color, whereas melanomas may evolve in size, shape, and color, and also exhibit symptoms like itching or bleeding. "A" = asymmetry, "B" = border, "C" = color, "D" = diameter, and "E" = evolving.

16. B) UVR causes DNA damage, resulting in mutations of key cancer genes

UVR causes multiple types of DNA damage, resulting in mutations of key cancer genes that control cell survival, proliferation, and differentiation. UVR includes both solar and artificial sources such as tanning beds. There are two main types of UV radiation: UVA and UVB. UVA passes deeper into the skin and causes indirect DNA damage. This is mediated by free radical formation and damage to cellular membranes. UVB is more carcinogenic than UVA. It is absorbed in the epidermis via sunburns and erythema, directly damaging DNA.

17. A patient with melanoma that has spread to distant points in the skin as well as to the brain is most likely diagnosed with which stage of melanoma?

    A. Stage I
    B. Stage II
    C. Stage III
    D. Stage IV

18. Which type of clinical trial focuses on developing improved imaging and laboratory tests?

    A. Screening
    B. Diagnostic
    C. Prevention
    D. Treatment

19. A nurse is looking for guidance on symptom management for a patient in a clinical trial. In which section of the clinical research protocol would the nurse find information about how symptoms can be managed while on the study?

    A. Study implementation
    B. Abstract
    C. Supportive care
    D. Eligibility assessment and enrollment

(See answers next page.)

17. D) Stage IV

Stage IV melanoma has metastasized to other places throughout the body, such as brain, lungs, liver, and distant points in the skin. Stage III has metastasized to nearby lymph nodes, lymph vessels, or skin. Stage II extends beyond the epidermis and is thicker than stage I and slightly more likely to metastasize. In stage II there is no evidence that melanoma has spread to the lymph tissues, lymph nodes, or body organs. In stage I, melanoma is no more than 1.0 mm thick with no evidence of metastasis to lymph tissues, lymph nodes, or body organs.

18. B) Diagnostic

Diagnostic clinical trials aim to develop better tests and procedures to identify and diagnose disease. Clinical trials that focus on screening assess for new and improved ways to detect disease and health conditions earlier in healthy people. Examples include obtaining of tissue samples, genetic testing, imaging tests, health histories, and physical examinations. Clinical trials that focus on prevention evaluate the effectiveness of ways to reduce the risk of developing disease or to prevent the disease from returning. Examples are lifestyle changes, medications, and vaccines. Treatment-focused clinical trials test new treatments or devices, new drug combinations, and new approaches to surgery and radiation treatment. These trials are categorized by phases.

19. C) Supportive care

The supportive care section provides guidance on managing the patient's symptoms while participating in the study. The study implementation section of a research protocol provides information about the study and treatment plan, such as the study design, how the intervention will be given, specimen collection, reasons a patient might be taken off a study, and other treatments a patient may or may not receive while on the study. The abstract section is a summary of the study background, objectives, eligibility, and design. The eligibility assessment and enrollment section provides further details on inclusion and exclusion criteria for joining a study. Other sections of a protocol include title page, table of contents, data collection, protection procedures, and drug information.

20. A nurse is reviewing a drug currently in a clinical trial and notes that there are 20 patients and that the goal of the trial is to determine the appropriate dosing schedule for the new drug. The nurse concludes that the drug is in which phase of the clinical trial?

    A. Phase 1
    B. Phase 2
    C. Phase 3
    D. Phase 4

21. A nurse is preparing to administer a patient's chemotherapy intravenously. The nurse dons a pair of chemotherapy-approved gloves and a low-permeability gown and uses an absorbency pad to transport the chemotherapy to the patient. After administration, the nurse disposes of the gloves, gown, and absorbency pad in the chemotherapy hazardous waste bin and washes their hands with soap and water. Which important piece of personal protection did the nurse omit?

    A. Face shield
    B. Double glove
    C. Hand sanitizer
    D. Double gown

22. What is the "A" in the ABCDEs of mole and melanoma recognition?

    A. Agile
    B. Asymmetrical
    C. Above
    D. Absolute

23. A patient with melanoma that is 0.5 mm thick and has not spread beyond the epidermis, lymph nodes, or lymph tissue would be diagnosed as having which stage of melanoma?

    A. Stage I
    B. Stage II
    C. Stage III
    D. Stage IV

(See answers next page.)

20. A) Phase 1
Clinical trials have three main phases, plus a fourth phase that takes place after the drug enters the market. Phase 1 studies are small—15 to 60 patients that all receive the same study drug. The goal of this phase is to determine a dose or dosing schedule that is safe for humans, called the maximum tolerated dose. In phase 2, the drug effectiveness is evaluated. Studies are larger than in phase 1, usually 100 to 300 patients, and include patients for whom the current standard of care is not effective for their diagnosis. The goal of phase 3 is to compare the new drug with the current standard treatment. Phase 3 studies include large numbers of people (hundreds to thousands), are conducted in multiple locations, and use randomization to assign patients to the control and treatment groups. Phase 4 occurs after the drug enters the market and becomes available to the general public. Evaluation of risks, benefits, and uses in real-life scenarios occurs, and this involves thousands of patients.

21. B) Double glove
Double gloving with chemotherapy-approved nitrile gloves is the standard of care for safe handling. A face shield is recommended when there is a risk of splashing, such as when emptying a urinal for someone receiving chemotherapy. The nurse washed their hands with soap and water, which is appropriate after removing gloves. Wearing a single low-permeability gown is sufficient practice; double gowning is not necessary.

22. B) Asymmetrical
The ABCDEs of melanoma is an acronym used for signs and symptoms of melanoma. "A" is for asymmetry. Normal moles are symmetrical in appearance, whereas melanomas tend to be asymmetrical. "B" = border, "C" = color, "D" = diameter, and "E" = evolving.

23. A) Stage I
In stage I, melanoma is no more than 1.0 mm thick with no evidence of metastasis to lymph tissues, lymph nodes, or body organs. Stage II extends beyond the epidermis and is thicker than stage I and slightly more likely to metastasize. In stage II, there is no evidence that melanoma has spread to the lymph tissues, lymph nodes, or body organs. In stage III, melanoma has metastasized to nearby lymph nodes, lymph vessels, or skin. Stage IV melanoma has metastasized to other places throughout the body, such as brain, lungs, liver, and distant points in the skin.

24. In assessing a patient with glioma prior to starting treatment, the oncology infusion nurse alerts the provider to which most concerning prognostic factor?

A. Age of 56 years
B. Karnofsky Performance Status Scale score of 55
C. Singular 2.5 cm brain tumor
D. Allergy to penicillin

25. The nurse evaluates a patient with multiple myeloma. Which finding is most significant for the patient's prognosis?

A. Hemoglobin 10.2 g/dL
B. Clonal bone marrow plasma cell percentage 70%
C. Creatinine 1.1 mg/dL
D. Beta-2 microglobulin 5.8 mg/L

26. A patient with breast cancer inquires as to why their cancer stage has been changed following mastectomy. The nurse's most precise response is:

A. "Pathologic information provides additional information for staging."
B. "Initial staging is only an estimate of disease burden."
C. "Once the tumor has been removed, the stage of the cancer is updated."
D. "The oncologist initially stages the tumor, but the surgeon finalizes the stage."

27. A priority teaching point for a nurse speaking to a patient about their new diagnosis of Barrett esophagus will be that the condition increases the risk of:

A. Squamous cell carcinoma of the esophagus
B. Adenocarcinoma of the esophagus
C. Squamous cell carcinoma of the throat
D. Adenocarcinoma of the throat

28. Which action will an oncology institution take to meet the Standards of Oncology Nursing Practice?

A. Enacting a quota regarding the ratio of male to female nurses hired
B. Requiring all nurses hired to have earned a bachelor of science in nursing degree
C. Individualizing nursing skill set standards based on the nurse's educational background
D. Asking the front-desk staff to provide each new patient with a welcome packet

(See answers next page.)

24. B) Karnofsky Performance Status Scale score of 55
A Karnofsky score of 55 is associated with poorer prognosis. Age of 56 years is not associated with poorer prognosis. While multiple metastases are associated with poorer prognosis, a singular metastasis is not. Allergy to penicillin does not have an influence on prognosis.

25. D) Beta-2 microglobulin 5.8 mg/L
A beta-2 microglobulin level of 5.8 mg/L classifies this patient as a stage III according to the International Staging System and indicates a poor prognosis with a median survival time of 29 months. Low hemoglobin and borderline-high creatinine levels are not particularly significant in assessing the patient's condition. A clonal bone marrow plasma cell percentage of 70% would be an expected finding in a patient with multiple myeloma.

26. A) "Pathologic information provides additional information for staging."
Pathologic information from intraoperative biopsies and specimens allows for pathologic staging. Initial, or clinical, staging is not an estimate of disease burden; rather, it is a staging based on radiographic findings alone. The stage of the cancer is not downgraded once a tumor has been removed. The oncologist, surgeon, and pathologist collaborate in staging.

27. B) Adenocarcinoma of the esophagus
Barrett esophagus increases the risk of adenocarcinoma of the esophagus 30 to 125 times. It is not associated with squamous cell carcinoma of the esophagus or the throat or adenocarcinoma of the throat.

28. B) Requiring all nurses hired to have earned a bachelor of science in nursing degree
The Standards of Oncology Nursing Practice recommends standardizing the criteria for nurse competency across an institution. Requiring all nurses to have a certain minimum level of educational training is one example of standardizing criteria. Enacting a quota based on sex would be inappropriate. Individualizing standards for nursing skill sets based on background would be counter to the Standards of Oncology Nursing Practice. A request for the front-desk staff to take a certain action does not fall under the umbrella of nursing standards.

29. Which term best describes a nurse's failure to turn on the bed alarm for a patient who is known to be at high risk for a fall?

A. Forgetfulness
B. Malpractice
C. False imprisonment
D. Negligence

30. A nurse notes that a colleague is displaying cynicism and exhaustion in the workplace and is expressing feelings of inefficacy. The nurse recognizes that this behavior is most likely due to:

A. Burnout
B. Compassion fatigue
C. Workplace violence
D. Apathy

(See answers next page.)

29. D) Negligence

Negligence is defined as substandard care based on the expected actions of a reasonable person. Although failure to turn on the alarm may result from forgetfulness, this does not adequately describe the impact on patient safety and care. Malpractice describes an action that deviates from professional standards. False imprisonment is holding an individual against their will.

30. A) Burnout

Exhaustion, cynicism, and feelings of inefficacy are characteristic of burnout. Compassion fatigue is similar but typically presents with distress. The colleague's presentation is not consistent with workplace violence or apathy.

Treatment Modalities

1. While discussing postsurgery instructions related to intraoperative radiation, the oncology nurse explains that the patient will:

   A. Be able to go back to work the same day as the procedure

   B. Need to schedule weekly radiation therapy visits

   C. Receive a single dose of radiation during the surgery

   D. Need a follow-up appointment for possible skin side effects from the treatment

2. A patient with leukemia preparing for hematopoietic stem cell transplantation will receive stem cells from the patient's sibling. This type of donation is known as:

   A. Autologous

   B. Allogeneic

   C. Anemic

   D. Autografted

3. Which organ systems require assessment and close monitoring for grading of graft-versus-host disease?

   A. Respiratory, skin, lymphatic

   B. Eyes, liver, renal

   C. Liver, skin, gut

   D. Heart, liver, gut

4. Human leukocyte antigen (HLA) markers determine the best possible source of stem cells for transplantation. Which donor is the best match?

   A. 2/10 HLA match from an unrelated donor

   B. 4/10 HLA match from a sibling donor

   C. 6/10 HLA match from an unrelated donor

   D. 8/10 HLA match from a sibling donor

(See answers next page.)

1. C) Receive a single dose of radiation during the surgery

Intraoperative radiation is a single dose of radiation given during the surgical procedure to radiate deep margins of tumors that cannot be resected. This is a major surgery with radiation treatment, so it is not reasonable to say that the patient can go back to work on the same day. Because this is a single-dose therapy, the patient will not need to schedule radiation therapy visits for this type of radiation, nor will they need a follow-up for skin side effects because the radiation is delivered to deep internal tissues of the tumor.

2. B) Allogeneic

Stem cells, bone marrow, and umbilical cord blood are allogeneic, regardless of whether they come from a related or an unrelated donor. Autologous donations come from the patient's own cells. Anemic refers to low red blood cell count. Autografted refers to the procedure of transplanting cells from the patient.

3. C) Liver, skin, gut

There is an important grading system for graft-versus-host disease involving the liver, skin, and gut systems. The liver is monitored by labs, especially bilirubin level. The skin is monitored by the percentage of rash covering the body. The gut is assessed by the volume of diarrhea per day. Respiratory, skin, lymphatic; eyes, liver, renal; and heart, liver, gut are not the right combination of organ systems for grading of graft-versus-host disease.

4. D) 8/10 HLA match from a sibling donor

A higher HLA match combined with a direct relationship to the donor is the best possible source. Any match below 6/10 is not considered optimal. Related donors are more ideal than unrelated donors, so an 8/10 HLA match from a sibling donor is a better option than a 6/10 HLA match from an unrelated donor.

5. A patient has been receiving nivolumab every 2 weeks for melanoma treatment. Baseline labs were within normal limits. During follow-up labs 2 months into treatment, results show an increased aspartate aminotransferase (AST)/alanine transaminase (ALT), 3× ULN (upper limit of normal). Bilirubin remains within normal limits. Which guideline would be most appropriate for the nurse to follow?

   A. Withhold nivolumab and repeat lab draws every 2 to 3 days until values normalize
   B. Discontinue nivolumab
   C. Begin corticosteroid therapy and continue nivolumab
   D. Continue nivolumab and increase lab monitoring

6. A patient is receiving bevacizumab treatment every 21 days and mentions an upcoming wrist surgery for carpal tunnel syndrome. The nurse anticipates that bevacizumab treatment will:

   A. Be held for 28 days before and 28 days after surgery, once wound has healed
   B. Not be modified; 21 days is appropriate after surgery once wound is healed
   C. Continue once the surgery site is well healed
   D. Be held for 28 days before surgery, resuming 21-day schedule after surgery

7. A nurse is preparing to administer the first dose of zoledronic acid to a patient recently diagnosed with bone metastasis. The physician order is for 4 mg intravenously (IV) every 4 weeks. The nurse is reviewing the patient's baseline labs and notes the following: creatine clearance (CrCl) 54, creatinine 1.0, and corrected calcium 9. The nurse confirms that which of the following is the most appropriate dose for this patient?

   A. Administer as ordered
   B. Administer 3.5 mg
   C. Administer 3.0 mg
   D. Administer 3.3 mg

8. A patient has been receiving zoledronic acid infusions for 3 months. The nurse is preparing to administer this month's infusion and, upon reviewing labs, notes the following: creatine clearance (CrCl) 55, creatinine 2.0, and corrected calcium 8.4. Which action would the nurse be prepared for now?

   A. Dose reduction
   B. Withholding the dose
   C. Increasing the dose back to baseline
   D. Administering a calcium infusion

(See answers next page.)

5. D) Continue nivolumab and increase lab monitoring

Transaminitis refers to increased liver enzymes and can be an adverse reaction during immunotherapy treatment. Elevated AST/ALT 3× ULN, when baseline labs were within normal limits and with no change in bilirubin, is considered grade 1 transaminitis. Nivolumab can be continued with more frequent lab draws per provider instructions. Grade 2 transaminitis criteria is AST/ALT 3–5× ULN with bilirubin 1.5–3× ULN. In grade 2, nivolumab should be withheld, labs should be repeated every 3 to 5 days, and prednisone should be considered. For grade 3 (AST/ALT >5–20× ULN and bilirubin >3–10× ULN) or grade 4 (AST/ALT >20× ULN or bilirubin >10× ULN), nivolumab should be permanently discontinued, and prednisone should be started.

6. A) Be held for 28 days before and 28 days after surgery, once wound has healed

Bevacizumab works by suppressing endothelial cell proliferation, vascular permeability, and angiogenesis. This can lead to impaired wound healing and complications such as necrotizing fasciitis. Treatment should not be given 28 days before or after 28 days after surgery and not until the wound has healed.

7. B) Administer 3.5 mg

To reduce the risk of acute kidney injury, baseline creatinine clearance should be obtained prior to initiating zoledronic acid. Four milligrams is the standard dose and safe to administer in patients with a baseline CrCl of >60. In patients with a baseline CrCl of 50 to 60, the appropriate dose is 3.5 mg. If CrCl is 40 to 49, dosing should be decreased to 3.3 mg. If CrCl is 30 to 39, dosing would be further decreased to 3 mg. Creatinine and corrected calcium are also monitored during zoledronic acid treatment to ensure adequate kidney function and calcium supply. This patient's creatinine and corrected calcium are within normal limits.

8. B) Withholding the dose

During treatment with zoledronic acid, creatinine should be monitored prior to each infusion and the dose withheld for signs of decreased renal function. Decreased renal function is defined as an increased creatinine of 0.5 mg/dL in patients with a normal baseline creatinine and an increase of 1.0 mg/dL in patients with an abnormal baseline creatinine. This patient's creatinine baseline was normal, and since this is an increase of 1.0 mg/dL, the appropriate action would be to hold this dose of zoledronic acid after discussion with the provider. This patient would also be instructed to increase their oral calcium supplement. Their calcium level is not low enough to warrant the need for a calcium infusion.

9. A patient receiving ipilimumab for 8 weeks reports having diarrhea for 3 days. Upon assessment, the nurse learns that the patient is having four to six stools a day along with cramping and urgency. Appropriate action from the nurse would be to:

   A. Confirm patient is taking antidiarrheals and suggest an increase
   B. Expect a delay in ipilimumab treatment to allow for corticosteroid treatment
   C. Refer patient to the provider for further gastrointestinal workup
   D. Expect discontinuation of ipilimumab for grade 4 diarrhea

10. Cyclin-dependent kinase (CDK) inhibitors, BRAF inhibitors, and epidermal growth factor receptor (EGFR) inhibitors are all examples of:

    A. Targeted therapy
    B. Chemotherapy
    C. Immunotherapy
    D. Hormone therapy

11. Which drug is fatal if given intrathecally?

    A. Cytarabine
    B. Bortezomib
    C. Methylprednisolone
    D. Methotrexate

12. All of the following are important components of safe blood administration EXCEPT:

    A. Use an 18-gauge or larger needle for infusion when transfusing red blood cells and platelets
    B. Administer irradiated blood components to allogenic hematopoietic stem cell transplant patients
    C. Use a leukocyte reduction filter and appropriate blood component set
    D. Transfuse red blood cells in less than 4 hours per unit from the time issued from the blood bank

(See answers next page.)

9. B) Expect a delay in ipilimumab treatment to allow for corticosteroid treatment

Immunotherapy-induced diarrhea is a common adverse event with checkpoint inhibitors such as ipilimumab, nivolumab, and pembrolizumab. Average onset of immune-induced diarrhea with ipilimumab is 7 weeks. Grade 1 diarrhea is classified as an increase of fewer than four stools per day over baseline, and patients should be monitored closely for any increase in symptoms. Antidiarrheals play a role; however, because the diarrhea is immunotherapy-induced, it can escalate quickly into a life-threatening situation if overlooked. Grade 2 is four to six stools a day over baseline and requires treatment delays along with corticosteroid administration for 4 to 6 weeks. Grades 3 and 4 include seven or more stools a day over baseline, incontinence, and hospitalization for complications of colitis. Treatment includes a higher corticosteroid dose and possible hospitalization for intravenous (IV) steroids and fluid administration.

10. A) Targeted therapy

Targeted therapies selectively target specific molecular pathways and include CDK inhibitors like ribociclib, BRAF inhibitors like dabrafenib, and EGFR inhibitors like lapatinib. Chemotherapy uses chemical agents to treat cancer and includes multiple classifications of drugs. Two examples are alkylating agents like bendamustine and antimetabolites like pemetrexed. Immunotherapy uses the body's immune system in the treatment of cancer and includes checkpoint inhibitors like nivolumab and monoclonal antibodies like denosumab. Hormone therapy interferes with levels of specific hormones in the body and is used in the treatment of cancers that are hormone sensitive. Examples include aromatase inhibitors like anastrozole and antiandrogens like enzalutamide.

11. B) Bortezomib

Bortezomib is fatal if given intrathecally. Cytarabine, methylprednisolone, and methotrexate are safe to administer intrathecally.

12. A) Use an 18-gauge or larger needle for infusion when transfusing red blood cells and platelets

Blood products may be infused in 24-gauge needles or larger. The smaller the gauge, however, the slower the flow rate and the higher the risk of clotting during transfusion. Patients who have undergone allogeneic hematopoietic stem cell transplantation require irradiated blood products to prevent the transfusion of leukocytes, which could result in a transfusion reaction. The use of a leukocyte reduction filter and appropriate blood component set reduces the number of leukocytes transfused to the patient, thus decreasing the incidence and severity of transfusion reactions. Packed red blood cells are initiated slowly for the first 15 minutes to monitor for initial transfusion reactions, with the remainder transfused over 1 to 3 hours per unit. Each unit must be transfused in less than 4 hours from the time of issuing from the blood bank to ensure stability.

13. A nurse is attempting to draw labs from a patient's implanted port and is unable to obtain blood return. After unsuccessfully flushing with normal saline using a push-stop method while pulling back for blood return, what action should the nurse take next?

    A. Reaccess the patient's port per policy
    B. Instill tissue plasminogen activator (tPA) with a provider order
    C. Ask the patient to change positions
    D. Continue push-stop method more forcefully

14. A patient with a newly implanted port comes in for their first chemotherapy infusion. Upon flushing the line, the nurse experiences resistance and is unable to obtain blood return. After the nurse asks the patient to change positions, the nurse is able to flush the line more easily when the patient looks down. When the patient looks back up, there is resistance again. What does this information indicate to the nurse?

    A. There is a fibrin sheath covering the end of the catheter tip
    B. Pinch-off syndrome (POS) is likely
    C. The catheter tip has migrated out of the superior vena cava
    D. Tissue plasminogen activator (tPA) administration is needed

15. A patient with a newly placed peripherally inserted central catheter (PICC) line arrives for their chemotherapy treatment. What action should the nurse take first prior to using the PICC line?

    A. Review chest x-ray to confirm placement
    B. Assess for blood return
    C. Attach tubing using aseptic technique
    D. Draw labs peripherally before initiating treatment

(See answers next page.)

13. C) Ask the patient to change positions

Signs of an occlusion in an implanted port are inability to push fluids and/or an inability to withdraw blood. The push-stop method causes a swirling action in the device to help maintain patency. The next step would be to ask the patient to change positions. Sit up, lie down, turn head and cough, and shrug shoulders are some examples that would help to break up the occlusion. If this does not work, reaccessing the port and instilling tPA are the next steps, per each institution's policies. Forceful pushing of fluids should be avoided to prevent catheter damage.

14. B) Pinch-off syndrome (POS) is likely

POS is when the catheter is pinched between the clavicle and the first rib, and mechanical friction over a prolonged period of time can cause catheter rupture or fracture. This happens during placement and could be avoided with proper placement by the surgeon. POS should be suspected when the catheter function changes with neck and arm movements, which occurs due to compression of the subclavian vein. When POS is suspected, the catheter should be promptly removed to avoid life-threatening complications such as catheter fracture and embolization of its fragments. When a fibrin sheath or line migration is suspected, flushing the line and obtaining blood flow are not dependent on head and neck positioning of the patient. tPA would be used if position change and flushing were unable to clear the line. The fact that this patient's flow was positional should alert the nurse to POS.

15. A) Review chest x-ray to confirm placement

PICC lines are inserted under ultrasound guidance with the distal tip of the catheter lying in the lower third of the superior vena cava. The catheter tip must be confirmed before initial use by ultrasound, fluoroscopy, or chest x-ray. Nurses should see that confirmation before using the PICC for the first time. Once placement is confirmed, the nurse would then check for blood return and draw labs through the line if needed rather than peripherally. Tubing is not attached until placement is confirmed, labs are drawn and reviewed, and treatment is initiated.

16. What test must be completed prior to each administration of bevacizumab?

  A. Urine protein
  B. Serum calcium
  C. Echocardiogram (ECHO)
  D. Serum magnesium

17. The nurse is reviewing a patient's chart and notes that the patient is receiving chemotherapy to reduce the size of a tumor before surgery can be performed. The nurse knows this is considered which type of therapy?

  A. Adjuvant therapy
  B. Intraoperative chemotherapy
  C. Neoadjuvant therapy
  D. Postoperative radiation

18. Docetaxel 75 mg/m² is ordered for a patient who has a body surface area (BSA) of 1.66 m². The patient weighs 60 kg and is 165 cm. The nurse calculates the docetaxel dose to be:

  A. 124.5 mg
  B. 46 mg
  C. 121.5 mg
  D. 75 mg

19. The patient's oncologist writes an order for paclitaxel 290 mg (175 mg/m²) intravenously (IV) over 3 hours. When the patient comes in for treatment, the nurse calculates the body surface area (BSA) at 1.7 mg/m² based on current height and weight. What is the appropriate action for the nurse to take?

  A. Administer 290 mg as ordered
  B. Administer 297.5 mg based on current height and weight
  C. Hold paclitaxel
  D. Refer to the institution's policy regarding dosing

(See answers next page.)

16. A) Urine protein

Bevacizumab treatment can lead to renal injury and proteinuria. Urine protein is tested prior to each dose by a urine dipstick analysis. Treatment should be delayed in patients with a 2+ or greater urine dipstick reading, and further assessment with a 24-hour urine collection is advised. Continue withholding bevacizumab if proteinuria is greater than or equal to 2 g/24 hr and resume dosing when proteinuria is less than 2 g/24 hr. Serum calcium and magnesium will be monitored routinely during treatment, but this is not always required prior to each dosing. ECHOs are important to monitor for patients receiving cardiotoxic drugs, as well as for anyone who experiences cardiac complications, but are not required prior to each dosing of bevacizumab.

17. C) Neoadjuvant therapy

Cancer treatment can include multiple methods, and surgery is the primary treatment with most solid tumors. When a treatment is done prior to surgery or another main treatment, it is called neoadjuvant therapy. For example, chemotherapy administration is done to reduce tumor size, allowing for a more conservative surgery. Adjuvant therapy is given after the primary treatment to lower the risk that the cancer will come back. Intraoperative chemotherapy is treatment given during surgery. Postoperative radiation is an adjuvant treatment, given after surgery to treat potential microscopic disease when conservative surgery was performed.

18. A) 124.5 mg

Most chemotherapeutic agents are dosed using the patient's BSA (m²). The BSA is a function of the patient's height and weight and can be calculated using formulas such as the DuBois & DuBois calculation. For BSA-dosed medications, it is important to compare the patient's current height and weight to the treatment plan when written. Adjustments may need to be made. The total dose of the agent is then calculated by multiplying the BSA by the ordered dose in mg/m², mcg/m², or g/m². In this case, the BSA was already calculated. $75 \times 1.66 = 124.5$ mg.

19. D) Refer to the institution's policy regarding dosing

Each institution has different policies in place for dose calculations and administration. Based on current height and weight, this patient's dose is 297.5 mg when calculated. Some institutions would have the ordered dose given unless there is a 5% or greater dose change when calculated. In this case, the difference is less than 5%. Other institutions may require exact dosing to be given based on patient's height and weight with each visit.

20. What is the best rationale for encouraging patients who are receiving immunotherapy to carry a wallet card?

    A. To be able to receive special treatment in public places like airports

    B. To alert providers in other care settings that immune-related side effects may require steroids

    C. To identify the patient as a cancer patient in case of an emergency

    D. To remember immunotherapy drug names because a wallet card has all of the important information

21. Which drug is fatal if given intrathecally?

    A. Vincristine

    B. Cytarabine

    C. Methotrexate

    D. Methylprednisolone

22. A patient is scheduled for their second dose of Rituxan. They did not experience any adverse reactions during the first infusion. According to the manufacturer's guidelines, at which rate may the Rituxan begin?

    A. 50 mg/hr

    B. 150 mg/hr

    C. 200 mg/hr

    D. 100 mg/hr

23. What is an example of oncoplastic surgery?

    A. Palliative debulking of a tumor

    B. Oophorectomy

    C. Breast reconstruction after mastectomy

    D. Cord compression surgery

24. Which patient would likely have better postsurgical outcomes?

    A. 27-year-old with a history of asthma and diabetes

    B. 52-year-old with sarcoma on the left second metatarsal

    C. 70-year-old with a history of lung cancer treated with chemotherapy and radiation

    D. 65-year-old with cachexia

(See answers next page.)

20. B) To alert providers in other care settings that immune-related side effects may require steroids

Immunotherapy wallet cards contain important information, such as the patient's diagnosis, the agent and drug name, start date, and provider information. Wallet cards are valuable for other providers to know that immunotherapy and chemotherapy are not the same thing, and that side effects may require steroids and a referral to the oncologist for care.

21. A) Vincristine

Vincristine is fatal if administered intrathecally. Cytarabine, methotrexate, and methylprednisolone are safe when administered intrathecally.

22. D) 100 mg/hr

According to the manufacturer's guidelines, a patient's first infusion of Rituxan should begin at 50 mg/hr and increase every 30 minutes by increments of 50 mg/hr, with a maximum rate of 400 mg/hr. Subsequent infusions, if no reaction occurs with the first dose, may begin at 100 mg/hr and increase every 30 minutes, with increments of 100 mg/hr to a maximum rate of 400 mg/hr. Interrupt or slow the infusion for reactions, and resume at half of the rate at which it was infusing when the reaction occurred once reaction symptoms resolve.

23. C) Breast reconstruction after mastectomy

Oncoplastic surgery improves appearance after an oncology surgery. Breast reconstruction after mastectomy (removal of breast) improves appearance. Palliative debulking of a tumor is a surgery that reduces discomfort when curative surgery is not possible. Oophorectomy is surgical removal of the ovaries and is a preventive procedure. Cord compression is an oncologic emergency surgery necessary to prevent or lessen the effects of a tumor on the spinal cord.

24. B) 52-year-old with sarcoma on the left second metatarsal

The 52-year-old patient with sarcoma, a type of solid tumor located on a bone in the foot, has no other comorbid conditions, which increases their chances of a better postsurgical outcome. The 27-year-old, 70-year-old, and 65-year-old patients have comorbid conditions. Cachexia is a nutritional deficiency and would be described as a comorbid condition.

25. What are significant considerations for treatment in patients older than 60 years prior to bone marrow transplant?

   A. Dose-reduced chemotherapy only

   B. Total body irradiation (TBI) only

   C. Same treatment as patients age 60 years and younger

   D. Dose-reduced chemotherapy, immunotherapy, and TBI

26. Processing peripheral blood stem cells (PBSCs) involves cryopreservation and dividing into smaller volumes called:

   A. Stem portions

   B. Aliquots

   C. Marrow fragments

   D. Segments

27. The nurse notes that a patient preparing for a bone marrow transplant describes a social lifestyle with lots of family members and friends. What will the nurse address as a primary risk factor in the plan of care for this particular patient?

   A. Electrolyte imbalance

   B. Impaired cardiovascular status

   C. Infection

   D. Fatigue

28. The nurse teaches a bone marrow transplant patient about the importance of isolation during treatment and why prophylactic medications are administered. The patient recalls having cytomegalovirus (CMV) in the past. The nurse would expect to teach about which medication?

   A. Trimethoprim–sulfamethoxazole (Septra, Bactrim)

   B. Ganciclovir (Cytovene)

   C. Voriconazole (Vfend)

   D. Amphotericin B (Fungizone)

29. The bone marrow transplant nurse expects which other treatments with high-dose cyclophosphamide (Cytoxan)?

   A. Psyllium fiber (Metamucil); docusate sodium (Colace)

   B. Diphenoxylate/atropine (Lomotil); clear liquids

   C. Mesna (Mesnex); intravenous (IV) hydration

   D. Fluconazole (Diflucan); saline mouth rinses

(See answers next page.)

25. D) Dose-reduced chemotherapy, immunotherapy, and TBI

Bone marrow transplant patients older than 60 years are specifically treated with dose-reduced chemotherapy, immunotherapy, and TBI. Patients younger than 60 years generally are given the full regimens of chemotherapy and immunotherapy without radiation. Dose-reduced chemotherapy only and TBI only are not options discussed for these patients.

26. B) Aliquots

PBSCs are harvested, cryopreserved, and divided into smaller volumes called aliquots. The nurse would transfuse the aliquots during the time of the transplant. Stem portions, marrow fragments, and segments are only smaller subset components of the peripheral blood cell and are not terms used in bone marrow transplant work.

27. C) Infection

Risk for infection is a primary concern for bone marrow transplant patients. The patient will likely want to continue their relationships, so the nurse will need to teach the patient about the risks. There is risk for electrolyte imbalance and fatigue in all patients undergoing treatment, but this patient's social history makes the potential for infection especially important to address. Risk for impaired cardiovascular status relates to cardiovascular history, which is not a risk factor for the patient at this time.

28. B) Ganciclovir (Cytovene)

Instructing the patient on the importance of isolation during bone marrow transplant treatment is vital to reduce the risk of potential infections and other complications. CMV is a herpesvirus infection that is latent in the body and can be reactivated by allogeneic incidence. Ganciclovir is an antiviral used to treat CMV. Trimethoprim–sulfamethoxazole is a combination of two antibiotics that prevents *Pneumocystis jirovecii* pneumonia. Voriconazole and amphotericin B are antibacterials used to prevent fungal infections.

29. C) Mesna (Mesnex); intravenous (IV) hydration

A side effect of cyclophosphamide is hemorrhagic cystitis. Mesna and IV hydration are required with this chemotherapy agent to offset the side effect. Psyllium fiber and docusate sodium are used to treat constipation. Diphenoxylate/atropine and clear liquids treat diarrhea. Fluconazole treats fungal infections, and saline mouth rinses may help oral tissue inflammation. None of these other treatments are viable for side effects of cyclophosphamide.

30. A patient with prostate cancer asks the radiation nurse why they need to undergo fiducial marker placement. The nurse educates the patient by responding:

A. "Fiducial markers are a safety measure to ensure the correct patient is receiving their treatment."

B. "Fiducial markers intensify the power of the radiation beams."

C. "Fiducial markers will be used to rule out recurrence during posttreatment surveillance."

D. "Fiducial markers act as a guide to ensure radiation is directed at the tumor even if your prostate moves."

(See answers next page.)

30. D) "Fiducial markers act as a guide to ensure radiation is directed at the tumor even if your prostate moves."
Fiducial markers are small metal beads inserted into the tumor site to guide radiation, particularly when the target tends to move, such as with the prostate. Fiducial markers are not meant to ensure that the correct patient is getting treatment, do not serve to intensify radiation beams, and are not used for surveillance.

Symptom Management and Palliative Care

1. Under Medicare guidelines, patients are eligible for hospice services when life expectancy is less than:

   A. 6 months
   B. 9 months
   C. 12 months
   D. 18 months

2. How might a nurse use the first "S" in the SPIKES mnemonic tool to help guide a difficult conversation for the patient and their family?

   A. Assess how much the patient understands about their current medical state
   B. Ask the patient how much information they would like to be shared with them
   C. Ask the patient who they would like to be with them when discussing their medical status
   D. Summarize the clinical information presented and develop steps for the next treatment plan

3. A patient with acute myeloid leukemia has transitioned to hospice care at home. The patient is no longer verbal, is struggling to swallow, and has clear secretions. The patient is moaning frequently and is visibly restless. When the patient's spouse requests pain management, which medication would the nurse determine to be most effective?

   A. Oral morphine tablet (MS Contin)
   B. Sublingual morphine solution (Roxanol)
   C. Hydromorphone suppository (Dilaudid)
   D. Oxycodone hydrochloride oral solution (Roxicodone)

4. A patient with small-cell lung cancer has been on hospice services for 2 weeks and is now verbalizing increased feelings of dyspnea. What will be the first-line therapy implemented to treat these symptoms?

   A. Nebulized morphine (MS Contin)
   B. Oral morphine (MS Contin)
   C. Oxygen therapy
   D. Oral lorazepam (Ativan)

1. A) 6 months
According to the Centers for Medicare & Medicaid Services, a patient is eligible for hospice services when they have a life expectancy of less than 6 months. A patient with a life expectancy of 9, 12, or 18 months would not be eligible for hospice services.

2. C) Ask the patient who they would like to be with them when discussing their medical status
The first "S" in the SPIKES mnemonic tool refers to the preparation of the setting for a difficult conversation. This includes who the patient would like to have in the room with them during that time. The "P" refers to the nurse's asking the patient's perception of their medical condition, which is done through inquiry and assessment. The "I" stands for invitation and speaks to how much information the patient wants presented. The second "S" stands for the nurse's summarizing the presented information and creating a plan for the next steps.

3. C) Hydromorphone suppository (Dilaudid)
Suppositories are a way for patients to experience pain relief when they are unable to take medications by mouth. Oral medications, including oral solutions, could pose a risk for aspiration or choking if the patient is unable to swallow. Sublingual medications, while quickly dissolved, still may present a risk because they cause increased oral secretions that need to be swallowed.

4. B) Oral morphine (MS Contin)
In this setting, the first-line therapy for dyspnea is opioids. Nebulized opioids have not been found to be beneficial in this setting. Oxygen therapy and oral lorazepam may be options to try if oral opioids are not successful.

5. A patient who practices Buddhism dies while in hospice at around midnight with the family present at the bedside. Understanding that cultural practices may affect how to proceed with posthumous procedures, how will the nurse ensure sensitivity to and respect for the patient and family?

A. Refer the family to the clergy of their choosing during movement of the body to the morgue

B. Allow the family to handle moving of the body based on cultural practices

C. Inquire as to which funeral home should be contacted to handle cultural preparation of the body

D. Ask the patient's family how they would like to proceed with their cultural practices

6. Which Palliative Performance Scale (PPS) level is a clinical indicator of impending death?

A. 100%

B. 50%

C. 30%

D. 10%

7. While discussing an upcoming chemotherapy treatment, the patient tells the nurse they are taking several herbal supplements in addition to their medications. Upon learning this information, the nurse will first:

A. Inform the patient that the use of all herbal supplements should be stopped during treatment

B. Obtain a list of herbal supplements and discuss possible interactions with chemotherapy

C. Explain that herbal supplements are not U.S. Food and Drug Administration (FDA)–regulated and are not recommended

D. Have the patient explain why they chose the supplements they are using and any benefits they have seen

8. The nurse suggests a referral for palliative care to the patient with advanced cancer because it improves overall quality of life. Which area also improves with access to early palliative care?

A. Family dynamics

B. Medicare benefits

C. Survival rate

D. Access to medical equipment

(*See answers next page.*)

5. D) Ask the patient's family how they would like to proceed with their cultural practices

When practicing culturally appropriate and sensitive care, the nurse will approach the family with a sense of inquiry on how to best help with cultural practices. In the Buddhist faith, the deceased's body should not be moved for several hours. This allows the patient's spirit to "leave without becoming confused." Moving the body immediately, even in conjunction with contacting a clergy member, may be inappropriate. The family would not be allowed to handle the moving of the body themselves; the nurse would help facilitate the movement for proper cultural preparations. Assuming a funeral home should be contacted immediately or first may be inappropriate.

6. D) 10%

A PPS level of 10% or lower indicates that the patient is in the end stages of life, with 0% meaning death has occurred. A PPS level of 100% indicates that the patient has normal activity level. A PPS level of 50% indicates an activity level of sit/lie, extensive disease, and normal or reduced intake; the patient may be conscious, drowsy, or confused. A PPS level of 30% indicates that the patient is unable to perform any activity, is completely bed bound, has reduced oral intake, and may be conscious or drowsy with or without confusion.

7. B) Obtain a list of herbal supplements and discuss possible interactions with chemotherapy

Some herbal supplements cause synergistic effects with chemotherapy, while others diminish the effects. Obtaining a list of herbal supplements and discussing it with the patient encourages an open dialogue for continued conversations and monitoring. More than half of cancer patients use complementary and alternative medicine, but one third do not report this to the healthcare team. Telling the patient to stop all herbal supplements may not be necessary, does not address the patient's reasons for taking supplements, and may discourage the patient from using other complementary therapies. Herbal supplements are not FDA regulated; however, some may be beneficial to specific patients, so there is no blanket recommendation against their use. Inquiring as to why the patient chose the supplements taken may open up dialogue but is not the first step to determining if the patient should continue.

8. C) Survival rate

Early palliative care improves rate of survival as well as alleviates most symptoms and decreases bouts of depression. Family dynamics and access to medical equipment are not affected by palliative care services. Palliative care is in place to aid the patient in comfort and does not address any form of benefits, including Medicare.

9. The nurse reviews prescriptions with the patient related to initiation of opioids for pain management. The patient will start oral long-acting morphine (MS Contin) 10 mg every 12 hours and short-acting morphine sulfate 15 mg every 4 to 6 hours as needed. The nurse discusses the potential for opioid-induced constipation. Which additional information would the nurse provide to the patient regarding this treatment?

   A. "It is important to add polyethylene glycol (Miralax) to your daily routine to avoid constipation."

   B. "Including methylcellulose (Metamucil) with your dietary intake will help reduce abdominal cramping."

   C. "You can use mineral oil as a laxative to promote stimulation of bowel movements."

   D. "Docusate (Colace) will stimulate bowel movements without cramping."

10. During a home hospice visit, the nurse finds that a patient with metastatic cancer is agitated and appears to be speaking to someone who cannot be seen. The patient is no longer oriented to person, place, or time. Which intervention is most appropriate?

    A. Reorient the patient to person, place, and time

    B. Administer haloperidol (Haldol)

    C. Administer lorazepam (Ativan)

    D. Place a consult to psychiatry

11. A patient with metastatic lung cancer reports increased shortness of breath. Vital signs show normal blood pressure (BP) and heart rate (HR), oxygen saturations of 96% on room air, and a temperature of 98.9°F (37.2°C). On assessment, the patient appears in no acute distress and denies pain. How will the nurse best address this patient's immediate need?

    A. Administer morphine (MS Contin)

    B. Begin oxygen via nasal cannula

    C. Obtain a chest x-ray

    D. Administer lorazepam (Ativan)

(See answers next page.)

9. A) "It is important to add polyethylene glycol (Miralax) to your daily routine to avoid constipation."

Polyethylene glycol (Miralax) is an osmotic laxative. Osmotic and stimulant laxatives are considered first-line treatment for opioid-induced constipation. Methylcellulose (Metamucil) is a bulk-forming agent and is contraindicated in advanced cancer patients because it requires increased water intake. Mineral oil and docusate (Colace) are stool softeners and would not benefit this patient because stool softening will not alleviate constipation.

10. B) Administer haloperidol (Haldol)

Delirium at end of life is very common, with symptoms including agitation, emotional lability, and hallucinations. Haloperidol (Haldol) is the best intervention for hyperactive delirium, as it blocks dopamine and can calm agitation and hallucinations. Reorienting the patient is not recommended when a patient has active hallucinations. Administering a benzodiazepine, like lorazepam (Ativan), can worsen delirium and cognitive impairment and is not recommended. A consult to psychiatry is not necessary for this patient because delirium in this patient's clinical scenario is not due to an active or suspected psychiatric disorder, but rather is due to end-of-life delirium, given that the patient is in hospice with metastatic cancer.

11. A) Administer morphine (MS Contin)

A patient's self-report of dyspnea is the red flag for assessment. A patient with metastatic lung cancer may have a tumor or an obstructive component affecting how the patient perceives the degree of dyspnea, despite adequate oxygen saturation. Opiates, typically morphine (MS Contin), are the initial intervention for managing dyspnea as they offer relief of tightness in the chest from anxiety related to the panic some patients feel when it seems as if they cannot breathe. Supplemental oxygen may not provide the best relief in all cases, but it can be used for comfort if the patient finds symptomatic improvement. A pleural effusion or infection may be contributing to the patient's shortness of breath and could be diagnosed on an x-ray, but relieving the patient's current complaint is the best first action given that the vital signs are normal. Benzodiazepines, like lorazepam (Ativan), can be helpful in managing concomitant anxiety with dyspnea, but opiates are the primary treatment for managing dyspnea.

12. During a palliative care consultation, the nurse sets up a private, quiet room for the consultation and ensures that the appropriate family members are present with the patient for the visit. Using the "SPIKES" mnemonic, what would the nurse say next?

    A. "Tell me your understanding of your cancer diagnosis."
    B. "I have some bad news to share with you regarding your recent CT scan results."
    C. "I can see that this information is difficult to hear and is very upsetting for you."
    D. "Are you the type of person who likes a lot of details, or do you prefer we talk about the big picture?"

13. A patient with metastatic colon cancer is receiving palliative care services and is trying to make a decision about enrolling in hospice. Which statement by the patient demonstrates their understanding of the difference between palliative care and hospice in the United States?

    A. "My doctor says I have a life expectancy of 6 months or less, so I qualify for hospice services."
    B. "Palliative care means that I am dying and do not have a long time to live."
    C. "I can continue my chemotherapy treatments while I am enrolled in hospice."
    D. "Being involved with the palliative care team means that I have to stop my chemotherapy treatments."

14. What is the most common side effect of radiation therapy (RT)?

    A. Fatigue
    B. Radiodermatitis
    C. Weight loss
    D. Myelosuppression

15. A patient receiving home hospice services complains of shortness of breath. What would be the best tool for the nurse to use to assess the patient's symptoms?

    A. FACES scale
    B. Respiratory Distress Observation Scale (RDOS)
    C. Numerical Rating Scale (NRS)
    D. Richmond Agitation-Sedation Scale (RASS)

(See answers next page.)

12. A) "Tell me your understanding of your cancer diagnosis."

The "SPIKES" mnemonic is often used in palliative care to effectively and empathetically communicate with patients and families. The letters of the acronym stand for Setting, Perception, Invitation, Knowledge, Emotion, and Strategy/Summary. Because the nurse has already established the appropriate setting by arranging for a private room and the presence of appropriate family, the next step is to address perception by having the patient explain their understanding of their diagnosis. Informing the patient of the need to share bad news addresses knowledge. By acknowledging the difficulty of the news and the effect it has on the patient, the nurse incorporates emotion. Asking the patient about the degree of desired detail incorporates invitation into the discussion.

13. A) "My doctor says I have a life expectancy of 6 months or less, so I qualify for hospice services."

As defined by Medicare, hospice is a benefit to patients with a life expectancy of 6 months or less. Palliative care is a broader term whose services are not exclusive to those at the end of life. One misconception in the United States is that palliative care is reserved for end-of-life care. Curative treatments are typically not covered as part of insurance hospice benefits, and thus would not continue for patients enrolled in hospice care. Patients enrolled in palliative care are able to continue curative or investigational treatments.

14. B) Radiodermatitis

Radiodermatitis, or radiation-related skin reaction, results from the delivery of ionizing radiation to the skin, causing cutaneous and subcutaneous lesions. It is the most common side effect of RT. Fatigue, weight loss, and myelosuppression are all side effects of RT but are not the most common.

15. C) Numerical Rating Scale (NRS)

When assessing the subjective report of dyspnea, the NRS is the most practical nursing assessment tool. The FACES scale is used to help patients express their pain level. The RDOS is used when patients cannot self-report due to changes in cognition. The RASS is used to evaluate a patient's agitation or sedation level.

16. A patient has a newly placed ostomy and is seeing it for the first time. The patient appears to be anxious. What nursing intervention would be most appropriate when starting the ostomy education process?

    A. Immediately begin removing the ostomy bag and dressing
    B. Explain how to obtain home ostomy supplies
    C. Measure the size of the stoma for proper flange placement
    D. Ask the patient what they want to learn first

17. A nurse is meeting with a patient to review pre-chemotherapy education and notes that the patient is taking opioids for cancer-related pain. Which nursing intervention would be most appropriate?

    A. Counsel the patient on the risk of addiction with opioid use
    B. Recommend a bowel regimen for prophylaxis and treatment of constipation
    C. Avoid discussing lifestyle modifications so as to not embarrass the patient
    D. Reassure the patient that opioid-induced constipation will be an issue

18. When educating a breast cancer patient undergoing lymph node dissection, the nurse would include which information in their education?

    A. Exercise should be avoided as it could make lymphedema worse
    B. Prophylactic massage of postsurgical scar tissue should be started immediately after surgery
    C. The risk of developing lymphedema is short term
    D. Compression garments should be used to manage lymphedema

19. Which of the following treatments has been proven to help with symptoms of anxiety, nausea, pain, and ability to cope after a mastectomy?

    A. Ondansetron
    B. Hydrocodone
    C. Acupuncture
    D. Massage

(See answers next page.)

16. D) Ask the patient what they want to learn first

The patient's anxiety may be relieved if the nurse asks them what they would like to learn about first. Immediately removing the ostomy bag and dressing would likely increase the patient's anxiety. Explaining how to obtain home ostomy supplies is important but is not the best thing to discuss first. Measuring the stoma is an important part of assessing the stoma but is not the first thing that should be discussed in the patient teaching moment.

17. B) Recommend a bowel regimen for prophylaxis and treatment of constipation

Constipation is a common symptom in patients with cancer, especially those taking opioids. Oncology Nursing Society (ONS) guidelines suggest that adult patients with cancer who are taking opioids should be counseled on lifestyle modifications to prevent and treat constipation, including increased fluid intake, exercise, and a high-fiber diet. Additionally, a prophylactic bowel regimen, including stool softeners and laxatives, should be offered. Controlling cancer-related pain is vital during cancer treatment, and opioid addiction should not be the focus.

18. D) Compression garments should be used to manage lymphedema

Incorporating active treatment interventions such as compression garments, exercise, and lymph massage are important components of preventing and managing lymphedema. Prophylactic massage, however, should not be initiated immediately after surgery to allow for wound healing. Patients who have had cancer-related surgery have a lifetime risk of developing lymphedema.

19. C) Acupuncture

Studies conducted on patients undergoing unilateral and bilateral mastectomies have shown that acupuncture can reduce the severity of anxiety, pain, and nausea and increase the ability to cope postoperatively. Ondansetron in prescribed for nausea, and hydrocodone is prescribed for pain. Massage may help with reduction of some of these symptoms, like anxiety and inability to cope, but it may affect nausea and pain due to physical touch and manipulation.

20. Which of the following recommendations would a nurse suggest to a patient who is experiencing nausea related to chemotherapy treatments?

    A. Eat spicy foods
    B. Skip dinner
    C. Sip liquids slowly throughout the day
    D. Eat foods low in calories and protein

21. The patient who would be advised against using peppermint oil as aromatherapy to help with side effects of cancer treatment is the patient who:

    A. Has nausea and vomiting
    B. Is taking anxiety medication
    C. Has sleep disturbances
    D. Has a history of atrial fibrillation

22. A patient presents to the infusion clinic for their chemotherapy infusion. Upon review of pre-chemotherapy labs, the nurse notes a total white blood cell (WBC) count of 1,600, polys = 48, and bands = 5. The absolute neutrophil count (ANC) parameters for chemotherapy administration are to proceed with treatment if ANC > 1,000. How will the nurse proceed?

    A. Proceed with treatment; ANC 1200
    B. Hold treatment; ANC 848
    C. Hold treatment; ANC 600
    D. Proceed with treatment; ANC 1124

23. Which of the following chemotherapeutic agents requires cardiotoxicity monitoring?

    A. Bortezomib
    B. Doxorubicin
    C. Gemcitabine
    D. Decitabine

(See answers next page.)

20. C) Sip liquids slowly throughout the day

Nausea can lead to dehydration, so it is important to educate patients to drink fluids throughout the day. Patients who are experiencing nausea should avoid spicy foods and instead eat bland food such as toast and crackers. They should not skip meals. It is important to eat small, frequent meals throughout the day, as nausea is more likely to occur on an empty stomach. Lastly, the patient should choose foods that are high in calories and protein.

21. D) Has a history of atrial fibrillation

While studies have shown that peppermint oil helps with symptoms of chemotherapy-induced nausea and vomiting, patients with a history of atrial fibrillation are advised not to use peppermint oil. The chemical constituents of peppermint oil stimulate the immune and nervous systems, which could affect heart rate and blood pressure. Peppermint oil has been shown to have positive effects on nausea, vomiting, stress relief, and sleep disturbances. Patients taking medication for anxiety and depression are advised to avoid lavender oil, not peppermint oil, as it could enhance the effects of the medication.

22. B) Hold treatment; ANC 848

ANC is calculated by adding the % neutrophils + % bands × WBC. 48 + 5 = 53. Convert to percentage = 53/100 = 0.53%. Multiply by total WBC = 0.53 × 1,600 = ANC = 848. ANC is below parameter, and treatment should be held.

23. B) Doxorubicin

Doxorubicin is in the anthracycline drug class. Anthracycline therapy is associated with an increased risk of developing heart failure, requiring cardiac monitoring such as echocardiograms for early recognition and intervention. Gemcitabine and decitabine are antimetabolites and do not routinely cause cardiac complications. Bortezomib is a proteasome inhibitor, and while it can lead to cardiac complications, routine cardiac monitoring is not required.

24. A nurse is educating a patient on myelosuppression precautions. The patient's hemoglobin (Hgb) = 10.2, absolute neutrophil count (ANC) = 1,650, and platelets = 50. Which of the following precautions would the nurse include in their education?

    A. Thoroughly wash raw fruits and vegetables before consuming
    B. Wash hands frequently and report any symptoms of infection
    C. Wear gloves while working in the garden
    D. Use a soft toothbrush and maintain skin integrity

25. Nonconventional therapies that are used in place of conventional treatments are known as:

    A. Complementary
    B. Alternative
    C. Integrative
    D. Spiritual

26. A patient receiving bortezomib is inquiring about complementary treatments to help with nausea, fatigue, and general well-being. Which of the following would the nurse caution the patient to avoid?

    A. Acupuncture
    B. Peppermint oil
    C. Green tea
    D. Guided imagery

27. Which of the following is the best rationale for the use of compression garments for a patient with lymphedema?

    A. To prevent accumulation of lymph fluid in soft tissue
    B. To help blood flow back to the heart
    C. To secure lymph nodes after mastectomy
    D. To identify the affected area

(See answers next page.)

24. D) Use a soft toothbrush and maintain skin integrity

The patient's labs are indicative of thrombocytopenia (<75,000 mm³). Precautions for this include maintaining skin integrity by using soft toothbrushes, using an electric razor instead of a straight edge, blowing the nose gently, and refraining from sexual activity that may compromise skin or mucous membrane integrity. Washing fruits and vegetables, washing hands, and wearing gardening gloves are neutropenic precautions and are discussed with patients with an ANC ≤1,500. A Hgb of 10.2 in someone undergoing chemotherapy does not require specific precautions; however, the patient would be considered anemic. Should the Hgb drop to 8 or less, transfusions are typically indicated. Patient education for anemia would include eating iron-rich foods and reporting worsening fatigue or shortness of breath.

25. B) Alternative

Alternative therapies are nonconventional therapies used in place of what is offered conventionally. Patients may choose these therapies if nothing is offered conventionally, if they have tried everything offered, or if what is offered conventionally does not align with their belief system. Examples include homeopathy and naturopathy. Complementary therapies are those that fall outside of conventional medicine and include acupuncture, herbal/botanical medicine, and mind–body and energy therapies. Integrative medicine combines complementary medicine with conventional treatment. Spiritual therapies are an example of complementary therapies and focus on beliefs and feelings about a sense of peace and connection to others, including spiritual healing and prayer.

26. C) Green tea

Complementary, alternative, and integrative therapies are used to enhance conventional therapies, as well as aid in symptom management and relief from side effects. Natural products should be used with caution as some can interfere with conventional medicine. For example, green tea should be avoided during bortezomib treatment as it can block the apoptotic effect of bortezomib. Acupuncture, peppermint oil, and guided imagery have all been shown to help with symptom management during cancer treatment; however, patients with atrial fibrillation should avoid using peppermint oil as it stimulates the nervous system and can affect heart rate and blood pressure.

27. A) To prevent accumulation of lymph fluid in soft tissue

Lymphedema occurs when there is an obstruction of the lymphatic system that causes accumulation of lymph fluid in interstitial spaces, resulting in swelling. This happens often in breast cancer after removal of lymph nodes, resulting in swelling to the arm on the affected side. Compression garments help by putting pressure on the area of swelling, helping it drain back through the lymph vessels, for recirculation back toward the heart.

28. Which of the following is true regarding fatigue?

    A. Exercise contributes to increased fatigue
    B. Fatigue often begins with cancer treatment
    C. Fatigue often resolves at the completion of treatment
    D. Adequate sleep and rest can help manage fatigue

29. A patient being treated with cetuximab for colon cancer has developed a facial rash. The nurse anticipates which of the following treatments?

    A. Cetuximab discontinuation
    B. Topical steroidal cream
    C. Intravenous (IV) antibiotics
    D. Diphenhydramine

30. At which time would a patient newly diagnosed with advanced cancer disease benefit MOST from a palliative care referral?

    A. Once the patient starts experiencing discomfort
    B. At the time of diagnosis
    C. During hospitalization for the disease
    D. Once they have 6 months or less to live

31. A patient has been given a Palliative Performance Scale (PPS) level of 10%. Their caregiver asks the nurse for advice on how they can best support the patient. The nurse recommends which of the following interventions?

    A. Offer frequent oral care for dry mouth
    B. Offer high-protein foods and fruits and vegetables
    C. Encourage normal activities of daily living
    D. Offer to help with end-of-life decision-making

(See answers next page.)

28. D) Adequate sleep and rest can help manage fatigue

Fatigue is a common complaint in cancer care. Ways of managing it include getting adequate sleep, rest, and relaxation and managing other symptoms. For example, fatigue may be more pronounced in someone with uncontrollable pain. Controlling pain will allow the patient to relax and sleep better, which will help with fatigue. Physical activity and exercise help with fatigue, not make it worse, as fatigue is not proportional to activity. Fatigue precedes and accompanies most malignancies, often being one of the first signs of disease. Unfortunately, fatigue does not always resolve at the completion of cancer treatment. Many cancer survivors complain of fatigue as a long-term side effect that affects quality of life.

29. B) Topical steroidal cream

Cetuximab is an inhibitor of estimated glomerular filtration rate (eGFR), with its most common side effect being an acneiform rash over the face, neck, upper chest, and back. It presents as papules and pustules, similar to acne, and usually does not require discontinuation. Oral antibiotics and topical steroidal cream are initiated to prevent discomfort and secondary skin infections. Diphenhydramine is given in the case of a histamine reaction. Acneiform rash associated with eGFR inhibitors is not due to a histamine response.

30. B) At the time of diagnosis

Palliative care offered at the time of an advanced cancer diagnosis is associated with improved quality of life, better symptom management, and cost savings if it is implemented early in the illness trajectory. Palliative care aims to improve discomfort; however, it can help prevent discomfort if implemented early enough. Palliative care can help prevent hospitalizations by identifying and treating discomfort and problems before they lead to hospitalization. Hospice care is offered when a patient's prognosis includes 6 months or less to live.

31. A) Offer frequent oral care for dry mouth

The PPS is a tool used to guide palliative and end-of-life care. There are five categories used for scoring: ambulation, activity level and evidence of disease, self-care, intake, and conscious level. It is scored from 0% to 100% in 10% intervals. A score of 0% is death. A patient given a PPS score of 10% or less is considered to have clinical signs of impending death. Mouth and lips can become dry during the dying process, and oral care helps to soothe the patient. Patients with a 10% level are not taking food or liquids, are bed bound, and are drowsy or unresponsive, requiring total care. This patient would be unable to discuss end-of-life decisions. A PPS score of 50% is given to a patient who mainly sits or lies in bed, is unable to do any work, and has extensive disease. These patients require considerable assistance with self-care, have normal or reduced intake, and have a level of consciousness ranging from full to drowsy, with or without confusion. A patient with a score of 100% has full ambulation capabilities, normal activities, no evidence of disease, full self-care and consciousness level, and full intake ability.

32. Which intervention would be appropriate to help alleviate secretions in a dying patient?

    A. Lower the head of the bed
    B. Apply a scopolamine patch
    C. Perform deep suctioning
    D. Perform chest percussion

33. Which intervention will be effective in managing excessive respiratory secretions as a patient begins the end-of-life stage?

    A. Increase oral and intravenous (IV) fluid intake
    B. Perform deep suctioning
    C. Keep patient lying flat in bed
    D. Administer atropine (Atropen)

34. A patient in hospice care has had an increase in secretions throughout the night that has not been improved by oral cavity suction. The patient's family is becoming increasingly upset with the "death rattle." What step will the nurse take to address this concern?

    A. Ask the family to step out of the room and perform deep suctioning on the patient
    B. Apply a scopolamine transdermal patch and continue to monitor secretions
    C. Explain to the family that the secretions are typical at this stage and will likely not respond to treatment
    D. Administer hyoscyamine (Levsin) orally every 4 hours and implement cough protocol

(See answers next page.)

32. B) Apply a scopolamine patch

A scopolamine patch is an anticholinergic agent that may be used for terminal secretions. Raising the head of bed is more effective than lowering, allowing secretions to drain. Deep suctioning is not recommended; however, shallow oral suctioning is appropriate. Chest percussion is not recommended.

33. D) Administer atropine (Atropen)

Studies are limited in the best interventions to manage secretions, but anticholinergic medications, like atropine (Atropen), can be helpful in drying the oral secretions when a patient is entering the end-of-life stage. Oral and IV fluid intake should be decreased or discontinued whenever possible, as they may make secretions worse. Deep suctioning is not generally effective and causes more distress to the patient and family. Repositioning the patient can help with secretion pooling and is a nursing intervention that can be safely tried.

34. C) Explain to the family that the secretions are typical at this stage and will likely not respond to treatment

The patient is producing type II secretions, which stem from the bronchi and are likely related to pulmonary pathology. While these secretions do not typically respond to treatment, educating the family on the pathophysiologic process may help ease their worries in the event treatment is not successful. Deep suctioning may cause more distress than benefit in a dying person, as it often causes gagging and may be painful. Since this patient is experiencing type II secretions that most often do not respond to treatment, pharmacologic intervention, such as a scopolamine transdermal patch or hyoscyamine (Levsin), would not be the best intervention because these forms of treatment are not intensive enough to break up secretions and alleviate symptoms in this stage of death and dying.

35. A patient hospitalized for failure to thrive has a body mass index of 15.5 on admission. The patient has oropharyngeal dysphagia related to advanced esophageal carcinoma and fails a swallow study. Advance directives state no artificial nutrition and name the spouse as healthcare proxy. The nurse is present while the provider reviews options for artificial nutrition versus palliative care with the patient and their spouse. The patient, who is alert, oriented, and appropriate throughout the hospital stay, maintains declination of artificial nutrition. The following day, the patient's spouse pleads for a feeding tube. The nurse explains:

   A. "I will request ethics and psychology consults to evaluate the patient's competency."
   B. "As the healthcare proxy, you have the final say. Can you sign the consent today?"
   C. "When your spouse loses capacity, you will meet with the provider again and complete the consent at that time."
   D. "Your spouse retains decision-making capacity; it is unethical to ignore treatment directives."

36. A patient with end-stage liver disease (ESLD) presents to the ED 3 days prior to trans-jugular intrahepatic portosystemic shunt (TIPS) placement with agitation, nausea, reduced urinary output, lower-extremity edema, worsening ascites, and jugular venous distention. There are no drug allergies. The best choice for single-dose postoperative pain medication in this patient is:

   A. Ketorolac injection, 30 mg intramuscularly once
   B. Tramadol 50 mg tablet, 1 tablet by mouth once
   C. Morphine injection, 5 mg intramuscularly once
   D. Fentanyl citrate solution, 25 mcg intravenous push once

37. A patient who recently ran out of oxycodone is exhibiting irritability, flu-like symptoms, insomnia, and diarrhea. The nurse would first:

   A. Assess for opioid withdrawal syndrome
   B. Provide loperamide as needed for diarrhea
   C. Educate the patient on alternative medications
   D. Refer the patient to counseling for opioid addiction

(See answers next page.)

35. D) "Your spouse retains decision-making capacity; it is unethical to ignore treatment directives."

The patient demonstrates competency to make decisions and is alert, oriented, and involved in daily activities. Additionally, the patient's declination of artificial feeding aligns with the advance directives. While an interdisciplinary approach, in which the nurse consults with ethics and psychology, can be valuable in such situations, it does not devalue a competent patient's decision. A healthcare proxy may not overrule a competent patient's treatment directives. The healthcare proxy may not make treatment decisions unless the patient lacks decision-making capacity. Further, it is unethical for the care team to make plans that diverge from a patient's treatment directives once that patient no longer has decision-making capacity.

36. D) Fentanyl citrate solution, 25 mcg intravenous push once

Fentanyl citrate is a good option for acute pain management in ESLD. No dose adjustment is indicated for a single-dose or infrequent bolus dosing. Nonsteroidal anti-inflammatory drugs, like ketorolac, are contraindicated in ESLD due to increased risks of bleeding, interference with diuresis, hepatotoxicity, and drug toxicity. Tramadol is a possible option in well-compensated ESLD, but this patient's presentation suggests decompensated disease. The patient's symptoms also suggest concomitant renal failure, which is common in ESLD. While morphine is an option for ESLD with preserved renal function, its use in patients with renal failure can lead to increased toxicity and respiratory depression.

37. A) Assess for opioid withdrawal syndrome

Irritability, flu-like symptoms, insomnia, and diarrhea are associated with opioid withdrawal syndrome. Neither providing loperamide nor educating the patient on alternative medications addresses the dependence on oxycodone that is the root cause of the patient's symptoms. The patient does not necessarily need referral for counseling because dependence and addiction are not synonymous.

38. An oncology patient presents to the ED with a temperature of 101.1°F (38.4°C) and an absolute neutrophil count of 463 cells/µL. Physician orders have been placed for intravenous levofloxacin and blood cultures. The nurse's next step is to:

    A. Call the pharmacy to check for drug–drug interactions
    B. Collect cultures from blood and other potential sites of infection
    C. Provide cool compresses for the patient's comfort
    D. Educate the patient's family on infectious disease protocols

39. A patient on immunotherapy treatment reports unintentional weight gain, sluggishness, and brittle hair and nails. What lab result should the nurse review first?

    A. Hemoglobin
    B. Potassium
    C. Thyroid-stimulating hormone
    D. Prolactin

40. A patient with chronic lymphedema of the right arm presents with erythema, warmth, and pain in the right arm. What is the priority nursing diagnosis?

    A. Impaired physical mobility
    B. Fatigue
    C. Risk of infection
    D. Altered body image

(See answers next page.)

38. B) Collect cultures from blood and other potential sites of infection

Neutropenia accompanied by fever strongly suggests infection. It is imperative to obtain cultures from all potential sites of infection, including blood, prior to initiating microbial therapy, because results of microbiology and sensitivity panels play a crucial role in selecting appropriate antibiotics. Evaluation of potential drug–drug interactions, patient comfort, and family education are important nursing roles, but they would not be next in the sequence of tasks.

39. C) Thyroid-stimulating hormone

Weight gain, sluggishness, brittle hair, and brittle nails are common symptoms of hypothyroidism, a possible immune-mediated effect, and could be diagnosed with a thyroid-stimulating hormone blood test. Abnormalities in hemoglobin, potassium, and prolactin do not typically cause these symptoms.

40. C) Risk of infection

Erythema, warmth, and pain are concerning for infection, particularly in a patient with lymphedema who is more prone to developing infections. While fatigue, impaired mobility, and altered body image may be a part of this patient's presentation, they are not the priority diagnoses.

Oncologic Emergencies

5

1. A patient who has been treated with whole-brain radiation complains of a new onset of headaches, nausea, confusion, and blurred vision. The nurse suspects that the patient has:

   A. Hypercalcemia
   B. Tumor lysis syndrome
   C. Superior vena cava syndrome
   D. Increased intracranial pressure (ICP)

2. A patient presents to the ED with nausea, vomiting, itching, and muscle cramps. They also complain of increased anxiety and weakness since their chemotherapy treatment yesterday. Lab results are as follows: uric acid 8.9 mg/dL, phosphorus 5.9 mg/dL, potassium 7.0 mEq/L, and corrected calcium 5.9 mg/dL. The nurse suspects which of the following oncologic emergencies?

   A. Superior vena cava (SVC) syndrome
   B. Tumor lysis syndrome (TLS)
   C. Hypercalcemia of malignancy
   D. Anaphylaxis

3. A patient was receiving their first dose of rituximab and developed symptoms of a hypersensitivity reaction. The reaction occurred while the rate of infusion was 100 mg/hr. The reaction resolved with supportive medications, and the provider ordered rituximab to resume. Which of the following is the appropriate rate to resume?

   A. 100 mg/hr
   B. 50 mg/hr
   C. 150 mg/hr
   D. 25 mg/hr

1. D) Increased intracranial pressure (ICP)

Since the patient had brain radiation, increased ICP should be suspected first. It occurs with an increase in brain tissue, blood, and/or cerebrospinal fluid in the intracranial cavity, resulting in nerve cell damage, permanent neurologic deficits, and death. Causes can include metastatic disease to the brain, blood clots, infection, metabolic disorders, and radiation to the brain. Signs and symptoms include headaches, nausea/vomiting, weakness, photophobia, blurred vision, confusion, and speech alterations. Hypercalcemia most often occurs from tumors metastasizing to the bone, hyperparathyroidism, vitamin D intoxication, and medications like diuretics. It would not be suspected first in a patient who has received brain radiation. Tumor lysis syndrome occurs after chemotherapy rapidly destroys cancer cells, and their cellular contents spill into the bloodstream, causing acute kidney injury. Superior vena cava syndrome results from compromised venous drainage of the head, neck, upper extremities, and thorax through the superior vena cava because of compression or obstruction of the vessel. Although it shares some similar symptoms with ICP, it would be suspected if the patient received chest radiation rather than brain radiation.

2. B) Tumor lysis syndrome (TLS)

The patient is presenting with signs and symptoms of TLS, which occurs when a large number of cancer cells are rapidly destroyed following treatment with an antineoplastic agent. This causes the cells to spill their contents into systemic circulation. It can manifest as electrolyte imbalances including hyperuricemia (≥ 8.0 mg/dL), hyperphosphatemia (≥ 0.5 mg/dL), hyperkalemia (≥ 6.0 mEq/L), and hypocalcemia (≤ 7.0 mg/dL). SVC syndrome occurs when blood flow through the SVC is blocked, resulting in breathing problems, lightheadedness, and swelling in the upper body. The patient's corrected calcium value indicates hypocalcemia, not hypercalcemia, of malignancy. Anaphylaxis is an acute reaction to a drug and would not occur the day after treatment.

3. B) 50 mg/hr

According to the prescribing information, interrupt or slow the infusion for reactions, and resume at half of the rate at which it was infusing when the reaction occurred, once reaction symptoms resolve. A patient's first infusion of rituximab should begin at 50 mg/hr and increase every 30 minutes by increments of 50 mg/hr, with a maximum rate of 400 mg/hr. Subsequent infusions, if no reaction occurred with the first dose, may begin at 100 mg/hr and increase every 30 minutes to a maximum rate of 400 mg/hr.

4. A newly diagnosed patient with non–Hodgkin's lymphoma and a high tumor burden is receiving their first infusion of rituximab. Which of the following is the patient most at risk for after rituximab infusion?

A. Hypercalcemia

B. Cardiac tamponade

C. Tumor lysis syndrome

D. Pneumonitis

5. Which oncologic emergency is a patient with severe hyponatremia most likely to have?

A. Hypersensitivity

B. Disseminated intravascular coagulation

C. Sepsis

D. Syndrome of inappropriate antidiuretic hormone (ADH)

6. A patient with metastatic lung cancer complains of a new onset of dull, localized lower back pain. The pain worsens when lying supine and when coughing. The patient states that they are feeling weak and unsteady on their feet. Which diagnostic study does the nurse anticipate will be performed first?

A. CT

B. PET

C. MRI

D. Myelography

7. A patient arrives for chemotherapy treatment with bevacizumab. Upon physical examination, the patient is complaining of nausea along with abdominal pain. Heart rate is 100, and the patient is pale. Which action should the nurse take?

A. Educate the patient on tips for nausea control during cancer treatment

B. Proceed with treatment as these are common side effects of bevacizumab

C. Hold the bevacizumab and contact the provider

D. Send the patient home, instructing them to call the provider if symptoms worsen

(See answers next page.)

4. C) Tumor lysis syndrome
Tumor lysis syndrome can occur in 12 to 24 hours in patients with non–Hodgkin's lymphoma and a high tumor burden. It occurs from cells rapidly lysing and releasing their cellular contents into circulation. Symptoms include acute renal failure, hypocalcemia, hyperuricemia, and hyperphosphatemia. Patients need to be educated on the importance of reporting any unusual symptoms to their providers.

5. D) Syndrome of inappropriate antidiuretic hormone (ADH)
Syndrome of inappropriate ADH is a condition in which ADH is inappropriately triggered despite normal fluid balance. The release of ADH causes hyponatremia and hypo-osmolality. Hypersensitivity is an immune-mediated response to a drug, and typically occurs during the infusion or shortly afterward. Hypersensitivity reactions are not linked to hyponatremia. Disseminated intravascular coagulation is a clotting disorder and is not linked to hyponatremia. Sepsis occurs when there is impaired regulation of the patient's response to infection.

6. C) MRI
A patient with metastatic lung cancer is at high risk for spinal cord compression due to metastatic spread of the disease, compromising the spinal cord integrity. Symptoms include dull, localized, or radiating pain that is worse when lying supine, coughing, or sneezing. As compression worsens, muscle strength, coordination, and sensory perception are impaired. The diagnostic study of choice is an MRI, where full visibility of the spine can be assessed for multiple sites of metastasis. CT scans are used when MRIs are unavailable. Myelography is used with or without CT when MRI is nondiagnostic. PET scans are sensitive and specific but less available than MRIs and should not be used alone for spinal cord compression diagnosis or treatment guidance.

7. C) Hold the bevacizumab and contact the provider
The nurse should suspect a bowel perforation, which is a life-threatening side effect of bevacizumab use. Initial symptoms include abdominal pain, nausea, vomiting, general ill appearance, and tachycardia. The nurse should hold the drug and contact the provider immediately. The patient should not be sent home, and continued bevacizumab treatment should not be administered until the diagnosis is confirmed and treatment is provided. Although educating patients on tips for nausea control during cancer treatment is always important, it is not the most appropriate action at this time because the patient is experiencing a potentially serious side effect that requires urgent care.

8. The patient most likely to develop the complication of bowel obstruction related to their disease is the patient with:

    A. Metastatic ovarian cancer

    B. Stage IV lung cancer

    C. Locally advanced breast cancer

    D. Liver cancer

9. The nurse is caring for a patient with ovarian cancer and a small bowel obstruction. The patient has a nasogastric (NG) tube in place. What is considered important nursing management for this patient?

    A. Have the patient lie flat in the bed for comfort

    B. Assess for pressure around the nostrils every shift

    C. Encourage drinking of fluids to prevent dehydration

    D. Instill air into the NG tube to check for placement

10. An older adult patient who has been receiving chemotherapy for colorectal cancer is admitted to the hospital with abdominal pain and distention, nausea and vomiting, and decreased appetite. The patient receives nothing by mouth and is receiving intravenous fluids. The patient develops sudden relief of the abdominal pain, followed by more severe pain and increased abdominal distention. What can the nurse expect the next step to be in the care of the patient?

    A. Surgery consult

    B. Total parenteral nutrition (TPN) for nutritional support

    C. Administration of corticosteroids

    D. Administration of a laxative

11. When do the symptoms of radiation pneumonitis most likely occur?

    A. During radiation

    B. Immediately after completion of radiation

    C. Prior to beginning radiation

    D. Within 4 to 12 weeks post radiation

(See answers next page.)

8. A) Metastatic ovarian cancer

Metastatic ovarian cancer is one of the most common cancers that cause disease-related bowel obstructions. Lung, breast, and liver cancer do not typically metastasize to the bowel and cause mechanical obstruction.

9. B) Assess for pressure around the nostrils every shift

It is important to assess the skin of the nostrils around the NG tube for pressure or breakdown every shift because invasive devices can cause skin breakdown. The area should be kept clean and dry. The head of the bed should be elevated 45 degrees to improve ventilation and prevent aspiration. The patient with a bowel obstruction receives nothing by mouth. Air should not be instilled into the NG tube because it can increase abdominal distention.

10. A) Surgery consult

Sudden relief of pain followed by more severe pain and increased abdominal distention are indicators of a bowel perforation. Surgery should be consulted immediately. TPN is not the next step in this case but may be a consideration after surgery to support nutrition. Corticosteroids and laxatives are not indicated in a bowel obstruction or perforation.

11. D) Within 4 to 12 weeks post radiation

The patient begins to develop symptoms of membrane formation, proliferation of pneumocytes, and sloughing of epithelium and endothelium within 4 to 12 weeks of radiation, which causes radiation pneumonitis. Radiation pneumonitis does not start during or prior to radiation. It is rare to experience radiation pneumonitis immediately after radiation therapy is completed.

12. A patient is receiving radiation therapy for treatment of lung cancer. The nurse monitors the patient for increased risk of developing radiation pneumonitis based on what factor?

    A. Concomitant administration of chemotherapy
    B. Inadequate nutrition
    C. Previous treatment with corticosteroids
    D. Metastatic disease

13. An adult patient who received chest radiation and chemotherapy has developed a cough and dyspnea, has an oxygen saturation of 88%, and now requires oxygen. What can the nurse expect the medical management of the patient to include?

    A. Additional radiation therapy
    B. Glucocorticoid therapy
    C. Antibiotics
    D. Chest percussion

14. The nurse is choosing a peripheral site to administer a vesicant chemotherapy to a patient. What site should the nurse choose to prevent extravasation?

    A. Antecubital region
    B. Area above wrist and below elbow
    C. Dorsal surface of the hand
    D. Wrist

15. While receiving vincristine, the patient exhibits swelling, redness, and a lack of blood return at the peripheral intravenous site. What treatment should the nurse expect to use?

    A. Cold therapy
    B. Dexamethasone
    C. Dexrazoxane and cold therapy
    D. Hyaluronidase and heat therapy

16. What is the mainstay of treatment for disseminated intravascular coagulation (DIC)?

    A. Intravenous immune globulin (IVIG)
    B. Platelet transfusion
    C. Treatment of the underlying cause
    D. Supportive care with pain medication

(See answers next page.)

12. A) Concomitant administration of chemotherapy

Concomitant administration of chemotherapy with radiation can increase the risk of radiation pneumonitis. Smoking history, poor performance status, age older than 60 years, and preexisting pulmonary or lung disease are also risk factors. Inadequate nutrition, corticosteroids, and metastatic disease do not increase the risk of developing radiation pneumonitis.

13. B) Glucocorticoid therapy

The patient is experiencing radiation pneumonitis. Glucocorticoid therapy is the treatment for radiation pneumonitis when symptoms are severe and impair gas exchange. This therapy should be tapered slowly to prevent a pneumonitis flare. Radiation therapy should be stopped with these symptoms. Antibiotics are not indicated because an infective process is not suspected. Chest percussion is not indicated; that process is used when mucus is found and needs to be moved from smaller airways into larger airways.

14. B) Area above wrist and below elbow

Veins above the wrist and below the elbow are larger than others. The antecubital region should be avoided due to flexion/movement. Veins in the hand and wrist tend to have minimal overlying tissue and are therefore not good choices for a vesicant.

15. D) Hyaluronidase and heat therapy

Vincristine is a vesicant that can cause cellular damage to the tissue. Hyaluronidase and heat therapy are the recommended treatments when this occurs. Dexamethasone is recommended for oxaliplatin extravasation. Dexrazoxane is recommended for adverse effects of daunorubicin, doxorubicin, epirubicin, and idarubicin. Cold therapy alone is recommended for adverse effects of dactinomycin, mitoxantrone, and paclitaxel.

16. C) Treatment of the underlying cause

The mainstay of treatment for DIC is treatment of the underlying cause, such as sepsis. IVIG is not effective in addressing DIC. Platelet transfusions and pain medications might be a consideration, but they are not the first choice of treatment to be considered.

17. A patient with disseminated intravascular coagulation (DIC) reports pain and heaviness in the right lower leg. The nurse's next step is to:

  A. Administer hydromorphone (Dilaudid) as needed

  B. Assess the patient for a deep vein thrombosis

  C. Encourage the patient to ambulate in the hallway

  D. Elevate the right leg for comfort

18. The nurse is performing an initial assessment of a patient admitted with disseminated intravascular coagulation (DIC). Which is the most important aspect of the patient's history to emphasize to the care team?

  A. The patient reports an allergy to morphine

  B. The patient has a strong family history of colon cancer

  C. The patient identifies as a Jehovah's Witness

  D. The patient consumes 1 to 2 beers/day

19. What are the main signs of syndrome of inappropriate antidiuretic hormone (SIADH)?

  A. Hyponatremia and hypo-osmolality

  B. Polyuria and hematuria

  C. Hypotension and tachycardia

  D. Hypernatremia and hyper-osmolality

20. Which cancer is most likely to cause syndrome of inappropriate antidiuretic hormone (SIADH)?

  A. Small cell lung cancer

  B. Non-small cell lung cancer

  C. Renal cell carcinoma

  D. Hepatocellular carcinoma

(See answers next page.)

17. B) Assess the patient for a deep vein thrombosis

DIC increases the risk of both bleeding and clotting. A patient reporting lower extremity pain and heaviness should be evaluated for venous insufficiency. Administering pain medication, encouraging the patient to ambulate, and elevating the leg would not be the most appropriate next steps.

18. C) The patient identifies as a Jehovah's Witness

Blood product transfusions are often necessary during the treatment of DIC. It is important to note that the patient is a Jehovah's Witness. Jehovah's Witnesses typically do not accept blood products, and this would be crucial to note when treating the patient. While it is important to assess medication allergies, family history, and social history, the patient's spiritual beliefs hold more significant implications.

19. A) Hyponatremia and hypo-osmolality

SIADH occurs when excessive antidiuretic hormone is released, resulting in fluid retention with hyponatremia and hypo-osmolality. Polyuria and hematuria, hypotension and tachycardia, and hypernatremia and hyper-osmolality are not typical indications of SIADH.

20. A) Small cell lung cancer

Neuroendocrine tumors, particularly small cell lung cancer, are most likely to cause SIADH. While SIADH can occur with non-small cell lung cancer, renal cell carcinoma, and hepatocellular carcinoma, it is far less common.

Psychosocial Dimensions of Care

1. A nurse is providing chemotherapy education to a patient who appears uninterested. What question could the nurse ask to better assess the patient's readiness to learn?

   A. What does the patient want to know?

   B. Does the patient have a preferred learning style?

   C. Does the teaching require modifications for education level?

   D. Are there religious or cultural practices affecting the learning process?

2. The spouse of a deceased patient is expressing feelings of guilt over the death and admits to constantly replaying the circumstances of the death in their mind. What other statement by the spouse would indicate to the nurse that they are experiencing complicated grief?

   A. "I understand that there is nothing I could have done differently."

   B. "I am feeling better after working with a grief counselor."

   C. "I am unable to return to work because I can't stop thinking about them."

   D. "I am lonely and I miss them terribly and have relied on my family and friends for support."

3. Which of the following personality traits pose the greatest risk for poorer coping strategies and prolonged emotional distress among cancer patients and their caregivers?

   A. Feelings of security

   B. High self-esteem

   C. Anxiety

   D. Low levels of negative thinking

4. A patient states, "I had the most beautiful long hair before I started chemotherapy, and now I look so ugly, and I am just so sad." This statement would be best followed by which response from the nurse?

   A. "Tell me more about what this is like for you."

   B. "You're almost done with treatment, don't give up."

   C. "Everyone loves you just the way you are."

   D. "It's just hair, and it will grow back."

1. A) What does the patient want to know?

All questions are important to consider when assessing readiness to learn. However, a patient who seems uninterested might not want to know any more than they have to. Some patients prefer to learn the basics, such as when to come for appointments and who to call if needed, while others want to learn every detail of their treatment plan. The nurse should not assume every patient wants to know the same things and must be aware that what the patient wants to know might be different from what the nurse thinks they want to know. Asking the patient what they already know and from what source is part of the assessment but is not the first choice for addressing the uninterested patient. Assessing the patient's educational background and level of literacy is also an important component of assessing readiness to learning, because adjustments may need to be made in how things are explained.

2. C) "I am unable to return to work because I can't stop thinking about them."

Complicated grief occurs when individuals have difficulty accepting the death of their loved ones and assimilating into life without the deceased. Manifestations include feeling guilty about the death, constantly replaying it in their mind, and imagining that they could have somehow prevented the death. Further symptoms include intense longing, emptiness and lack of meaning in life, intrusive thoughts of the deceased that interfere with functioning, and recurring thoughts of wanting to join the deceased. Understanding that nothing could have been done differently, feeling better after working with a counselor, and being lonely and relying on friends are normal responses to grief and the dying process and do not indicate complicated grief.

3. C) Anxiety

Personality plays a role in how an individual grieves, internalizes the grief, and integrates understanding about the loss of a loved one. Certain personality traits are correlated with poorer coping strategies and prolonged emotional distress. Examples include anxiety, insecurity, low levels of self-esteem, and high levels of negative thinking.

4. A) "Tell me more about what this is like for you."

For this patient, hair loss has altered their body image. Altered body image is used to describe a state of disturbance in which the person's changed body image has affected the way they experience their usual sense of self. Communication strategies for nurses to best support patients include using exploratory and empathetic phrases, rather than premature reassurance or cheerleader-type encouragement. Altered body image can affect quality of life, leading to anxiety, depression, and social withdrawal. Using exploratory and empathetic communication allows the patient to process their feelings, rather than shutting down further communication.

5. A nurse is discussing sexuality concerns with a patient undergoing radiation and chemotherapy. Which statement from the patient would indicate to the nurse that more education on intimacy during cancer treatment is needed?

   A. "I use vaginal lubrication to avoid pain during intercourse with my partner."
   B. "My partner understands that I need more time to become stimulated."
   C. "We use condoms so that my partner doesn't come in contact with chemotherapy chemicals."
   D. "We avoid having sex because I am scared my partner will be affected by the radiation in my body."

6. A patient is preparing to return to work after completion of their cancer treatment. How can the nurse support the patient with employment concerns?

   A. Encourage the patient to take their pain medication so they can perform their prior work duties
   B. Encourage the patient to take more time off if they are worried about not being able to fully perform their job
   C. Remind the patient that employers are obligated to make accommodations to allow for return to work
   D. Refer the patient to a financial counselor to discuss concerns and evaluate the need to return to work

7. A patient with cancer receiving palliative care reports increasing worry, difficulty sleeping, and fatigue. Which medication should the nurse expect to be prescribed for this patient?

   A. Diphenhydramine
   B. Citalopram
   C. Ondansetron
   D. Docusate sodium

8. A patient's spouse admits feelings of sadness and fear and sleep disturbances. They worry constantly that their spouse "isn't strong enough to beat this." The nurse identifies this person to be experiencing which of the following?

   A. Bereavement
   B. Anticipatory grief
   C. Mourning
   D. Prolonged grief

(See answers next page.)

5. D) "We avoid having sex because I am scared my partner will be affected by the radiation in my body."

Radiation therapy from an external machine does not make the patient radioactive or harm their partner in any way. Patients undergoing radiation need this reassurance to feel safe maintaining closeness with their partners. Chemotherapy and radiation therapy can cause decreased vaginal lubrication and hypoactive arousal. Condom use is recommended during the first week following each chemotherapy administration to prevent exposure to medications excreted in body fluids.

6. C) Remind the patient that employers are obligated to make accommodations to allow for return to work

The Americans with Disabilities Act prohibits discrimination based on disability and requires employers to make accommodations. Reminding the patient of this can help relieve concerns about being unable to fully perform their job. Nurses need to understand the financial impact of cancer care and support the patient's return to work if they choose to return. Also, returning to work may help in improving a survivor's quality of life and should be encouraged.

7. B) Citalopram

The patient is exhibiting symptoms of generalized anxiety. Citalopram is a selective serotonin reuptake inhibitor and is effective in the palliative care of cancer patients for management of generalized anxiety. Diphenhydramine is an antihistamine that would not typically be used for generalized anxiety. Ondansetron is an antiemetic that would be prescribed for a patient complaining of nausea. Docusate sodium is a stool softener to be prescribed for a patient experiencing constipation.

8. B) Anticipatory grief

Anticipatory grief is a psychologic and somatic response to an anticipated loss. It includes symptoms such as sadness, inability to sleep, fear of life without their loved one, not wanting to be alone, and feelings of anger or guilt. Bereavement is the period during which grief and mourning occur after suffering a loss. Mourning is the outward expression of grief through death and bereavement rituals (e.g., wearing black clothes). Prolonged grief is identified as severe grief, causing significant distress and disability, lasting beyond 6 to 12 months after a loss.

9. Which of the following should a nurse be aware of when assessing a patient's and their caregiver's emotional response to living with cancer?

   A. Anticipatory grief and thoughts of suicide are the most common psychologic symptoms experienced by individuals with serious illness

   B. The ability to differentiate between depression and normal sadness will be clear

   C. Caregivers are at an increased risk for cardiovascular disease and stroke

   D. Having a support system does not affect overall emotional well-being

10. Which of the following cancer survivors is at greatest risk for financial burden and food insecurities?

    A. A 24-year-old who just graduated from college

    B. A 69-year-old who is on Medicare

    C. A 60-year-old who is looking ahead to retirement

    D. A 30-year-old who is working for a large corporation

11. When a patient in end-stage cancer expresses worry about leaving their family in a financial bind, with which first step will the nurse most appropriately address the patient's concern?

    A. Listen attentively to ensure the patient feels heard

    B. Contact the provider for an order for antianxiety medication

    C. Refer the patient and family for psychosocial counseling

    D. Provide information on community support resources

12. A clinical assessment tool used to assess concerns related to finances, psychosocial well-being, and impaired relationships in patients with cancer and their caregivers is:

    A. Zarit Burden Interview

    B. Caregiver Burden Scale

    C. Preparedness of Caregiving Scale

    D. Beck Depression Inventory

(*See answers next page.*)

9. C) Caregivers are at an increased risk for cardiovascular disease and stroke

Caregivers are at an increased risk for cardiovascular disease, stroke, and death. The most common psychologic symptoms experienced by individuals with a serious illness are anxiety and depression. Grief, anticipatory grief, and thoughts of suicide do occur; however, they are not the most common. The difference between normal sadness and depression is not always clear and can require assessment by a psychologic professional for appropriate interventions. Patients who lack a support system or have an inadequate support system may experience more emotional suffering compared with patients who have supportive systems in place. With any psychologic assessment, the nurse should listen well and practice advanced communication skills that will help the suffering patient and their caregivers feel heard and understood.

10. A) A 24-year-old who just graduated from college

Younger cancer survivors are at a greater risk for financial burden because they may not have had the opportunity to accumulate wealth and may still need to repay student loans. They face a longer future of healthcare costs due to increased risk of secondary cancers, psychologic distress, toxicities, and pain. It is likely that younger cancer survivors may have to sacrifice their economic needs, such as retirement planning, and reduce expenses for necessities such as housing and food. Older cancer survivors are more likely to have higher income and supplemental private insurance in addition to Medicare.

11. A) Listen attentively to ensure the patient feels heard

The most appropriate first step to addressing the patient's concern is to listen to the patient to provide a sense of calmness and trust so the patient feels heard. Once the patient has been allowed to express their concerns and worry, the nurse can then make the needed decisions to best provide the patient with resources and assistance.

12. A) Zarit Burden Interview

The tool used that includes both patient and caregiver in assessing for burdens related to finances, psychosocial well-being, and relationship impairment is the Zarit Burden Interview. The Caregiver Burden Scale is used to assess anxiety and burdens related to caring for a patient with cancer or other terminal illness. The Preparedness of Caregiving Scale is an assessment tool to determine the ability of the caregiver to provide needed assistance without feeling overwhelmed and burdened. The Beck Depression Inventory is used to assess the patient's level of depression.

13. A primary risk factor that will be monitored for in adolescents undergoing chemotherapy is:

    A. Comorbid diseases
    B. Altered body image
    C. Altered sexual identity
    D. Decline in treatment adherence

14. The nurse is conducting a follow-up postoperative assessment of a patient who recently underwent limb-sparing surgery for intramedullary sarcoma. The patient has also been undergoing chemotherapy and radiation treatment. The patient is noted to be cachectic and has Grade 1-2 alopecia. While assessing the surgical wound, the patient notes mild neuropathy and a lack of appetite but no nausea or vomiting. The patient, does, however, appear to be very conscious of the alopecia and is constantly trying to cover up their head. When creating the nursing care plan for this patient, which outcome would be a priority?

    A. The patient will exhibit decreased emotional distress and maintain an individualized support system
    B. The patient will identify appropriate food choices and nutritional guidelines to reach a 3-lb weight increase by the next visit
    C. The patient will optimize functional status to include roles and relationships as well as social interaction
    D. The patient will identify contributing factors for altered body image, adaptive coping strategies, and overall improved body image

15. While providing discharge instructions to an older adult patient on nutrition needed for weight gain, the nurse goes through a list of foods to consume and a list of foods to avoid. The patient states that they understand, and the patient is discharged. At the follow-up evaluation, the patient has lost 4 lb. What has most likely occurred?

    A. Due to their age, the patient is cognitively unable to understand the instructions provided
    B. The nurse did not ensure that the patient understood by asking the appropriate follow-up questions
    C. A family member or caregiver was not present to ensure total understanding of the instructions provided
    D. The nurse failed to determine if there are any barriers to communication and how the patient learns

(See answers next page.)

13. B) Altered body image

One of the highest risk factors in adolescents undergoing treatment for cancer is altered body image due to loss of hair, change in shape and structure of the body, and change in ability to function without becoming fatigued. Adolescent patients should be monitored for signs of depression and anxiety related to altered body image. Comorbid diseases may be seen in adolescents but are not commonly a high risk that would be monitored for. Likewise, altered sexual identity is not specific to treatment for cancer and would not increase the risks in adolescents. Most adolescents will adhere to treatment regimens even if they do not feel well, so this is not an increased risk factor.

14. D) The patient will identify contributing factors for altered body image, adaptive coping strategies, and overall improved body image

The priority intervention and related goal is to address the psychosocial aspect of care and the patient's self-consciousness regarding the loss of hair. While nutrition and diet would be a second important goal, altered self-image can exacerbate the psychologic issues related to appetite as well as increase the risks for depression and suicide. At this visit, the patient does not appear to be in distress but could benefit from individualized psychosocial support; this, however, is not the priority for the patient. Individualized support and care will also help the patient to optimize functional status as well as social interaction but is also not the priority at this time.

15. D) The nurse failed to determine if there are any barriers to communication and how the patient learns

Determining if there are barriers to communication such as hearing or visual impairment as well as the patient's learning style is important when providing education to a patient because people may best learn visually, aurally, or kinesthetically. Some patients would rather have a lot of big-picture information while others need information broken down into smaller components. This patient may not be a visual, aural, or global learner and therefore would need information provided in another format or written down. The patient should not automatically be considered cognitively impaired due to their age. While asking appropriate follow-up questions is important, if there is a communication barrier that is not recognized, then this will not be useful in determining if the patient truly understands. Having a family member or caregiver present is wise; however, if communication barriers and learning styles are not recognized, this will be ineffective.

Part II
Practice Exam and Answers With Rationales

Practice Exam

1. The nurse is reviewing the results of a patient's screening colonoscopy. A finding of which histologic type of polyp would be most concerning?

    A. Villous
    B. Tubular
    C. Tubulovillous
    D. Multiploid

2. Which is the most common histologic type of colorectal cancer?

    A. Squamous
    B. Carcinoid
    C. Adenocarcinoma
    D. Lymphoid

3. Which is the best description of the role of the oncology nurse navigator (ONN)? The ONN:

    A. Helps the patient access healthcare and overcome barriers in the system
    B. Partners with multiple institutions to recruit patients to sites
    C. Assists with specific high-needs patients diagnosed with cancer
    D. Acts as a social worker but has nursing knowledge and experience

4. Which organization establishes standards for oncology nursing practice?

    A. Oncology Nursing Society (ONS)
    B. American Nurses Association (ANA)
    C. The Joint Commission (TJC)
    D. American Nurses Credentialing Center (ANCC)

5. Which practice does not reflect quality nursing documentation?

    A. Nursing interventions documented at the end of shift
    B. Changes in patient's condition or response documented
    C. Events and interventions documented in sequential order
    D. Documentation including objective nursing judgment

6. The benefit of a nursing licensure compact is that it allows nurses to practice in:

    A. Any state regardless of where they obtained their nursing license
    B. A different state for a 3-month grace period before needing to apply for state licensure
    C. Multiple hospitals simultaneously
    D. Select states regardless of where they obtained their nursing license

7. Which is the best assessment tool for evaluating whether a nurse is experiencing compassion fatigue?

    A. PLISSIT
    B. PRoQOL
    C. CAGE
    D. ABC

8. What is the role of The Joint Commission?

    A. To oversee nursing procedures among institutions
    B. To investigate accusations of malpractice in the inpatient setting
    C. To develop standards for nursing education programs
    D. To provide accreditation to healthcare organizations

9. A nurse is caring for a patient who refuses blood products due to religious beliefs. The nurse does not share this view but respects the patient's right to choose. The nurse is adhering to which principle of healthcare ethics?

    A. Justice
    B. Autonomy
    C. Beneficence
    D. Nonmaleficence

10. The practice of providing patients with adequate information represents:

    A. Paternalistic advocacy
    B. Simplistic advocacy
    C. Consumer advocacy
    D. Existential advocacy

11. What is the primary purpose of obtaining certification in oncology nursing?

    A. It instills confidence in the public that the nurse has the proper education and training
    B. It instills confidence in the nurse when practicing in the oncology setting
    C. It justifies the salary paid to oncology nurses
    D. It identifies holes in current nursing education programs

12. A patient who is terminally ill with pancreatic cancer expresses a wish to die and inquires about euthanasia. What is the nurse's most appropriate first step?

    A. Inform the patient that their advance directive will need to be edited
    B. Reinforce the notion that life is worth fighting for
    C. Assess for psychiatric disorders or coexisting pain
    D. Refer the patient to a program in a state where euthanasia is legal

13. A nurse's current duties in the hospital include taking vital signs and assisting patients to the bathroom. These duties run counter to the recommendation in the Institute of Medicine's (IOM) 2011 report *The Future of Nursing: Leading Change, Advancing Health* that nurses should:

    A. Practice to the full extent of their education
    B. Participate in all aspects of patient care
    C. Be involved in policy and procedure development
    D. Have a bachelor's of science degree in nursing as minimum education requirement

14. What is the minimum number of oncology practice hours required to become an Oncology Certified Nurse (OCN)?

    A. 500 hours within the past year
    B. 500 hours within the past 2.5 years
    C. 1,000 hours within the past 2.5 years
    D. 1,000 hours within the past 5 years

15. A nurse is leading a quality improvement project in the oncology department. Which type of research article will be most compelling as supporting evidence for the project?

    A. Systematic review of qualitative studies
    B. Single-site randomized clinical trial
    C. Case study
    D. Systematic review of randomized clinical trials

16. Which of the following is considered the weakest type of research evidence to support a change in practice?

    A. Systematic review of randomized clinical trials
    B. Cohort studies
    C. Systematic review of qualitative studies
    D. Single-site qualitative study

17. The approximate overall incidence rate of severe hypersensitivity reactions to chemotherapy and biotherapy agents is:

    A. 25%
    B. 15%
    C. 5%
    D. 10%

18. Which communication tool can the nurse use to assist a palliative care patient to set goals for care and decision-making?

    A. SPIKES
    B. FACES
    C. MMSE
    D. PQRST

19. A nurse is caring for a patient who is beginning chemotherapy treatment with a taxane agent, paclitaxel (Taxol). The nurse will monitor the patient for signs of hypersensitivity, including:

    A. Atrial fibrillation
    B. Hypotension
    C. Incontinence
    D. Ataxia

20. The chemotherapy agent that has the highest potential for severe hypersensitivity reactions is:

    A. Anthracyclines
    B. Asparaginases
    C. Dacarbazines
    D. Antimetabolites

21. The nurse is caring for a patient with breast cancer who has a central line. The patient reports fatigue, muscle twitching, and heart palpitations. Upon assessing the patient, the nurse finds that the patient is hypertensive and bradycardic. The nurse interprets these symptoms as:

    A. Central line infection
    B. Hypercalcemia
    C. Urinary tract infection
    D. Bowel obstruction

22. The nurse recognizes that a rapid onset of breathing difficulties and anxiety in a patient receiving monoclonal antibodies can be a symptom of:

    A. Rhabdomyolysis
    B. Anaphylaxis
    C. Hypertension
    D. Malignant hyperthermia

23. The nurse knows that radiation-associated solid tumors are common secondary malignancies in patients with cancer that appear:

    A. 10 or more years after radiation treatment
    B. 5 years after radiation treatment
    C. Less than 6 months after radiation treatment
    D. Between 1 and 3 years after radiation treatment

24. Hypercalcemia is a life-threatening complication that presents in what percentage of cancer patients?

    A. 50% to 75%
    B. 1% to 5%
    C. 10% to 30%
    D. 30% to 50%

25. The nurse is incorporating the role of the patient's key caregiver while developing an end-of-life care plan. The nurse:

    A. Asks the patient to select a key caregiver of the same gender as the patient
    B. Teaches care to the key caregiver and asks them to convey that knowledge to secondary caregivers
    C. Takes into account cultural characteristics that may affect the key caregiver's role
    D. Suggests that the patient select someone who is unrelated to prevent family discord

26. A nurse is planning bereavement care for the family of a patient who is receiving hospice care in the home. The plan should include:

    A. Arranging for the patient's body to be removed from the home immediately
    B. Cleaning and dressing the patient's body
    C. Enlisting the family's help in removing equipment
    D. Ensuring that the family is not at the patient's bedside at the moment of death

27. The provider has prescribed hydromorphone and transdermal fentanyl for a patient experiencing breakthrough pain. The nurse explains to the patient that:

    A. Hydromorphone is a long-acting analgesic, and transdermal fentanyl is a rapid-release analgesic
    B. Hydromorphone is stronger than transdermal fentanyl
    C. Hydromorphone is a rapid-release analgesic, and transdermal fentanyl is a long-acting analgesic
    D. Transdermal fentanyl does not work well without concomitant use of hydromorphone

28. The hospice patient is experiencing spiritual distress. Which member of the interdisciplinary team would best help the patient?

    A. Volunteer
    B. Chaplain
    C. Oncologist
    D. RN

29. When the patient receives emetogenic treatment, the nurse knows that:

    A. It is all right for the patient to drive home
    B. They should follow up with the patient within 24 to 48 hours after the patient returns home
    C. They should reassure the patient that nausea and vomiting are not a serious concern
    D. The patient may develop hypervolemia

30. Nonpharmacologic methods to alleviate pain:

    A. Are greatly effective as the only method of pain relief
    B. Are most often used with pharmacologic methods to relieve pain
    C. Should never be used for severe pain
    D. Have a longer-lasting effect than pharmacologic methods

31. The nurse knows that a patient with advanced colorectal cancer is most likely to have metastases to the:

    A. Spleen
    B. Liver
    C. Lungs
    D. Stomach

32. Suspicious testicular masses discovered with ultrasound will be:

    A. Biopsied in situ
    B. Monitored for 3 months for enlargement
    C. Followed up with radical inguinal orchiectomy
    D. Examined more thoroughly with a scan

33. What intervention would be most appropriate for a young adult with altered body image?

    A. Encourage slowly acknowledging and including changes into daily activities and social relationships
    B. Provide the patient and family with community resources to support family dynamics
    C. Allow the patient to express concerns and reassure them things will return to normal after treatment
    D. Educate the patient on developing scheduled time for self-affirming statements to improve self-esteem

34. A patient who prefers to learn how to self-administer medications by demonstrating the action is what type of learner?

    A. Visual
    B. Global
    C. Kinesthetic
    D. Analytical

35. The nurse overhears a patient newly diagnosed with end-stage colon cancer tell their spouse, "It's not that serious," and indicating that "chemotherapy will take care of it." The patient is exhibiting the coping mechanism of:

    A. Denial
    B. Suppression
    C. Displacement
    D. Rationalization

36. The nurse is conducting a follow-up postoperative assessment on a patient who recently underwent a hysterectomy with bilateral salpingo-oophorectomy due to Stage IIIA1 (T1-N1-M0 or T2-N1-M0) ovarian cancer. The patient has also been undergoing chemotherapy and radiation treatment, which has led to cachexia, Grade 2 alopecia, and extreme fatigue. During the assessment, the patient begins to cry, stating that their spouse, who is the primary caregiver, has started to become angry and agitated with the patient. What steps will the nurse take to best address this patient's concerns?

    A. Refer the patient for psychosocial counseling and support
    B. Conduct a needs and abilities assessment of the patient's family and caregiver
    C. Request an order from the provider for corticosteroid medication for the patient
    D. Counsel the patient on proper nutrition and educate on food choices to ensure weight gain

37. An example of existential advocacy in patients with cancer includes:

    A. Providing information and supporting the patients' decisions
    B. Ensuring patients have adequate and accurate information
    C. Doing something on behalf of another for their own good
    D. Ensuring that patient beliefs are accepted and supported

38. A patient recently diagnosed with esophageal cancer is admitted to the ED with alcohol toxicity. The patient's family member reports that the patient has been consuming more alcohol and antidepressant medication since their diagnosis. Friends and family have attempted intervention multiple times with no success. Once the patient is stabilized, what step would the nurse take to address the primary need in this patient?

A. Provide support services for family and friends
B. Admit the patient to an inpatient rehabilitation facility
C. Assess the patient's stress and coping mechanisms
D. Educate the patient and family on appropriate coping skills

39. When working with a patient and their family, the nurse discusses the needs of the patient after discharge from the hospital, which will involve assistance with activities of daily living such as meal preparation and bathing. Several family members express concerns about providing personal care. What action will the nurse take first to meet the patient's needs?

A. Refer the family to counseling and support for caregivers
B. Assess the family as a whole and the ability to collectively care for the patient
C. Provide the patient with a list of community resources to provide care
D. Recommend the patient be admitted to a palliative care facility

40. A patient diagnosed with breast cancer is being seen for a follow-up visit in which possible bilateral mastectomy will be discussed. Information regarding the procedure was sent home with the patient at the last visit, and the patient has a list of questions and concerns, primarily around the implications of surgery on sexual identity. How can the nurse best address the patient's concern?

A. Provide information on breast reconstruction services
B. Refer the patient to a support group for breast cancer survivors
C. Schedule a consultation with a plastic surgeon to discuss postsurgical options
D. Encourage the patient to seek counsel within their religious organization

41. When a patient who has suffered from a long, difficult battle with colon cancer dies, the spouse appears to be in the accepting phase of grief. The spouse has most likely experienced what type of grief previously?

A. Inhibited
B. Delayed
C. Anticipatory
D. Disenfranchised

42. Complications from disease progression such as anxiety can impact the patient by:

    A. Exacerbating pain
    B. Causing constipation
    C. Increasing caregiver burden
    D. Increasing risk for drug misuse

43. A patient diagnosed with Stage II (T2, N0, M0) bladder cancer reports extreme fatigue, loose bowel movements, and a rash on the lower abdomen. The patient has been undergoing trimodal therapy with mitomycin-C and fluo-rouracil (5-FU) and has lost 8 lb over the past 6 weeks. The patient's family is concerned for the safety of the patient due to recent comments about "ending it all" and not being able to "take it anymore." What priority intervention would the nurse implement for this patient?

    A. Contact the provider for dosage adjustment
    B. Refer for nutritional support and counseling
    C. Refer for psychiatric admission and evaluation
    D. Alert the provider for an order of corticosteroids

44. When a patient recently diagnosed with terminal cancer begins to display signs of depression, the nurse would:

    A. Refer the patient for psychiatric evaluation
    B. Encourage the patient to discuss feelings
    C. Report to the provider for medication orders
    D. Reassure the patient that support is available to them

45. A young adult patient is undergoing preoperative assessment for hysterec-tomy with bilateral salpingo-oophorectomy. The patient is single, lives alone, and works full-time as a teacher. The patient does not have any children and has decided to harvest eggs for the future. When preparing the patient for postsurgical care needs and discharge information, which primary focus in care will the nurse address?

    A. Postoperative care and support
    B. Resources for fertility preservation
    C. Counseling for altered body image
    D. Access to community services and supplies

46. How can a loss of personal control impact outcomes in a patient diagnosed with cancer?

   A. Self-efficacy will be impacted and therefore will result in the patient's nonadherence to treatment

   B. Adjustment to disease is facilitated by the patient's emotional response to the disease

   C. Feelings of anxiety and stress are replaced by feelings of sadness and desperation

   D. Optimism and motivation are decreased, which impedes the patient's ability to meet treatment goals

47. The best definition of palliation in patient care is:

   A. Use of high-dose opioids to alleviate pain

   B. Alleviation of bothersome symptoms

   C. Decision to forego life-saving treatments

   D. Care for a patient with more than 6 months' expected survival

48. An older hospitalized patient with chronic cancer-related pain is diagnosed with opioid-induced constipation. What medication order will the nurse expect?

   A. Methylcellulose (Citrucel) 500 mg caplets, four caplets three times daily while taking opioids

   B. Methylnaltrexone (Relistor) injection, 8 mg subcutaneously every other day for 10 days

   C. Naltrexone (Vivitrol) injection, 380 mg intramuscularly (IM) once per week for 4 weeks

   D. Naloxone (Narcan) injection, 0.04 mg (40 mcg) intravenous (IV) push once daily for 3 days

49. The nurse completes assessment of a patient with cancer who suffers daily breakthrough pain. The nurse modifies the patient's care plan to include:

   A. Putting the patient's affairs in order

   B. More frequent visits from family and friends

   C. Adjuvant, nonpharmacologic comfort measures

   D. Time for the patient to spend in life review

50. A patient with end-stage renal disease (ESRD) elects to discontinue dialysis. Four days later the patient stops responding to outside stimuli and has blood pressure of 66/32 mmHg, pulse of 36 beats/min, and respiratory rate of four breaths/min. As-needed medications ordered include alprazolam (Xanax) 1 mg intravenous (IV) every 4 hours for agitation and morphine sulfate 2 mg IV every 2 hours for pain. Which encounter best demonstrates the principle of double effect?

   A. The patient begins pulling at the IV tubing. Agitation continues 30 minutes after alprazolam 1 mg IV is given, so the nurse contacts the ordering provider for additional options.
   B. The nurse knows the patient must feel terrible and administers 2 mg morphine sulfate IV every 1 hour to ease the transition.
   C. The patient becomes combative. The nurse administers lorazepam 2 mg IV because the patient has not yet required a dose today.
   D. The patient transitions into active dying and begins gasping respirations. This activity interferes with the roommate's sleep, so the nurse administers a dose of morphine sulfate.

51. What is considered the cardinal sign of increased intracranial pressure (ICP)?

   A. Brain metastases
   B. Papilledema
   C. Headaches
   D. Peripheral edema

52. Which statement is true regarding advance directives?

   A. Advance directives threaten patient autonomy
   B. It is not the nurse's responsibility to speak to the patient about advance directives
   C. Nurses report a lack of time and knowledge to help patients with advance directives
   D. Advance directives do not improve the likelihood that the patient will receive their chosen end-of-life care

53. What symptom is evident in more than 95% of patients with spinal cord compression (SCC)?

   A. Tachycardia
   B. Pain
   C. Horner syndrome
   D. Rash

54. A patient being treated for breast cancer has an Ommaya reservoir and complains of morning headaches and nausea, vomiting, and weakness. The nurse would be concerned with which oncologic emergency?

    A. Anaphylaxis

    B. Increased intracranial pressure

    C. Superior vena cava syndrome

    D. Spinal cord compression

55. Which type of cancer is responsible for most cases of superior vena cava syndrome (SVCS)?

    A. Breast cancer

    B. Colon cancer

    C. Lung cancer

    D. Sarcomas

56. A patient with lung cancer complains that their shirt collars are very tight and appears to have facial swelling and visible veins. Which oncologic emergency would the nurse be concerned about?

    A. Anaphylaxis

    B. Increased intracranial pressure (ICP)

    C. Superior vena cava syndrome (SVCS)

    D. Spinal cord compression (SCC)

57. A patient with an Ommaya reservoir who has breast cancer is admitted to the hospital with headaches, nausea, vomiting, and weakness. What would the nurse do to immediately manage this oncologic emergency?

    A. Administer preordered pain medication to the patient

    B. Assess the patient's device for proper placement

    C. Put the patient on bed rest and elevate head of bed 30 degrees

    D. Consult neurology for removal of the patient's Ommaya reservoir

58. A patient being treated for sarcoma with metastasis to the lung complains of shortness of breath after walking, racing heart, chest pain, and restlessness. Which oncologic emergency will the nurse be concerned with?

    A. Cardiac tamponade

    B. Increased intracranial pressure (ICP)

    C. Superior vena cava syndrome (SVCS)

    D. Spinal cord compression (SCC)

59. What symptom found in patients with cardiac tamponade is associated with a decrease in blood pressure of more than 10 mmHg during inspiration?

    A. Papilledema
    B. Pulsus paradoxus
    C. Pericardial friction rub
    D. Jugular vein distention

60. Which oncologic emergency could result directly from tumor invasion of the vertebrae?

    A. Pneumonitis
    B. Tumor lysis syndrome
    C. Spinal cord compression
    D. Superior vena cava syndrome

61. What treatment modality involves administration of drugs that act directly on specific molecules within the cancer cell?

    A. Chemotherapy
    B. Radiation therapy
    C. Targeted therapy
    D. Immunotherapy

62. The patient with cardiac tamponade is scheduled for a pericardial window. The nurse reviews orders and sees an anesthesia consult. The nurse will expect the anesthesiologist to make which statement?

    A. "I do not recommend this procedure because any anesthetic preparation will be too dangerous."
    B. "Local anesthesia is preferred because anesthesia with intubation may cause hypotension and cardiac arrest."
    C. "Anesthesia with intubation is preferred because the airway remains open and can protect cardiac function."
    D. "Local anesthetic for pericardiocentesis only will be recommended to limit the risk for hypotensive crisis."

63. Which routine intervention prevents occlusions in vascular access devices?

    A. Dressing changes
    B. Flushing
    C. Administering diphenhydramine
    D. Extravasation

64. Classifications of immunotherapies include:

    A. Checkpoint inhibitors and chimeric antigen receptor therapy
    B. Poly(ADP-ribose)polymerase (PARP) and proteasome inhibitors
    C. Epidermal growth factor receptor (EGFR) and human epidermal growth factor receptor 2 (HER2)
    D. RTK and TKIs

65. Companion diagnostics are used to evaluate molecular, genetic, and chemical characteristics using a companion assay to:

    A. Predict outcomes and monitor response
    B. Identify patients most likely to benefit from therapy
    C. Determine scheduling, dosages, and discontinuation of treatment
    D. Determine cell growth and proliferation

66. The nurse knows that the patient admitted for a particular chemotherapy needs to have a central venous catheter. What type of vascular access device will likely be used?

    A. Peripheral catheter
    B. Peripherally inserted central catheter
    C. Midline catheter
    D. Intrapleural catheter

67. The patient understands what chemotherapy entails but does not know what the provider means when they mention adding a targeted therapy medication. Which explanation would the oncology nurse begin with?

    A. "It's actually very similar to chemotherapy, except it is given before radiation to boost its effects."
    B. "Your medication is called paclitaxel (Taxol), and it works with your chemotherapy to get rid of your cancer."
    C. "Your medication, bevacizumab (Avastin), prevents your cancer cells from growing."
    D. "Your medication, mesna (Mesnex), allows us to safely use your chemotherapy drug, ifosfamide (Ifex)."

68. Biotherapies are made from what type of organisms?

    A. Augmented
    B. Living
    C. Dead
    D. Biosimilar

69. A patient being treated for breast cancer has recent scans showing tumor progression from Stage III to Stage IV with indications of metastasis to the lung. Which explanation describes what has most likely occurred?

    A. Immunotherapy has failed to eradicate tumors
    B. Tumor escape has allowed any tumor cells to progress
    C. Cytokines have failed to stimulate and regulate the immune system
    D. Monoclonal antibodies harbor specific tumor markers preventing eradication

70. What intervention will the nurse implement to achieve positive patient outcomes for a patient receiving biotherapy?

    A. Monitor for hypoglycemia
    B. Educate patient on adverse events
    C. Monitor for hypertension
    D. Educate patient on input and output

71. The oncology nurse is providing education to a patient who will undergo autologous chimeric antigen receptor therapy (CAR-T). What information will the nurse include?

    A. Blood from a donor will be modified and infused into the patient
    B. The patient's red blood cells are modified to attack cancer cells
    C. Blood cells need to be reprogrammed with tumor antigen receptors
    D. The procedure will take place over the course of a 24-hour period

72. What type of immunotherapy conditions the cancer patient's immune system to generate its own response to tumor growth?

    A. Chimeric antigen receptor therapy
    B. Checkpoint inhibitors
    C. Vaccinations
    D. Proteasome inhibitors

73. Trastuzumab (Herceptin) interferes with human epidural growth factor receptor 2 (EGFR-2), which is involved with tumor growth and progression. Which therapy is it an example of?

    A. Chemotherapy
    B. Immunotherapy
    C. Targeted therapy
    D. Radiation therapy

74. Which type of therapy treats cancer through the use, stimulation, augmentation, or suppression of immune system cells?

   A. Chemotherapy
   B. Immunotherapy
   C. Targeted therapy
   D. Radiation therapy

75. The nurse used the patient's power injectable implanted port to complete chemotherapy infusions. The patient will now go for a CT scan. The patient asks why the nurse is not removing the implanted port needle. What is the nurse's response?

   A. "You are right, I'll remove the port needle before your CT."
   B. "The needle will remain in place until your chemotherapy is completed."
   C. "Your port can be used for the high infusion pressure of CT contrast."
   D. "The radiology technician will remove the needle and insert a peripheral catheter for the CT contrast."

76. VEGF is an example of a:

   A. Chimeric antigen receptor T cell
   B. Checkpoint inhibitor
   C. Chemotherapeutic agent
   D. Target molecule

77. The nurse cares for a patient receiving chemotherapy and radiation therapy for renal cancer. A care plan for the patient includes:

   A. Weekly weights
   B. Limiting fluid intake
   C. Weekly vital signs
   D. Monitoring for fluid volume excess

78. The nurse asks the patient who has been prescribed opioids if they are constipated. The patient replies "No, I do not have to strain when I have a bowel movement. My last bowel movement was 4 days ago." The nurse replies:

   A. "It sounds like you are not constipated."
   B. "One bowel movement a week is sufficient."
   C. "It is fortunate that you do not have diarrhea."
   D. "I will need to complete an abdominal assessment."

79. A patient with impaired integument will be receiving care in the home from family members. The nurse teaches the family to:

   A. Turn the patient twice daily
   B. Assess the patient's skin twice daily
   C. Briskly massage the impaired skin areas
   D. Use an air or water mattress on the patient's bed

80. A female patient status post radical cystectomy asks the nurse if the surgery will affect sexual function. The nurse explains:

   A. "Sexual dysfunction is likely because of damage to the nerves."
   B. "Don't worry, you will still be able to have children."
   C. "Your sexual function will improve now that the cancer is gone."
   D. "Your partner might not find you as attractive because of the surgery."

81. An oncology patient presents to the ED with a temperature of 101.1°F (38.4°C) and an absolute neutrophil count of 463 cells/µL. Provider orders have been placed for intravenous levofloxacin and blood cultures. The nurse's next step is to:

   A. Call the pharmacy to check for drug–drug interactions
   B. Collect cultures from blood and other potential sites of infection
   C. Provide cool compresses for patient comfort
   D. Educate the patient's family on infectious disease protocol

82. Which intervention will the nurse include in the care plan for the patient with motor impairment?

   A. The patient will perform active range of motion on affected limbs 3 to 4 times a day
   B. The patient will use assistive devices when ambulating
   C. The nurse will reposition the patient in bed every 4 hours
   D. The nurse will always ambulate the patient

83. *RAS* is an example of a:

   A. Tumor suppressor gene
   B. Proto-oncogene
   C. Caretaker gene
   D. Chromosome translocation

84. Alterations in the *BRCA1* and *BRCA2* genes are examples of:

   A. Carcinogens
   B. Germline mutations
   C. Somatic mutations
   D. Breast cancer

85. The process of creating new blood vessels from existing ones is known as:

   A. Cell proliferation
   B. Energy metabolism
   C. Angiogenesis
   D. Oncogenetic division

86. An alteration that occurs in one location, or one base pair of DNA, is known as a:

   A. Point mutation
   B. Germline mutation
   C. Genetic defect
   D. Single switch

87. Which organ acts as a filter for blood cells and aids in fighting antigens in the blood?

   A. Thymus
   B. Spleen
   C. Thyroid
   D. Liver

88. The spread of cancer from its original site in the body to distant organs is called:

   A. Metastasis
   B. Stage III disease
   C. Perineural invasion
   D. Extracapsular spread

89. Which vaccine is recommended for the prevention of cervical cancer?

    A. Hepatitis B
    B. High-risk human papillomavirus (HPV)
    C. Shingles
    D. Influenza

90. What type of barriers do bile, tears, and perspiration represent?

    A. Physical
    B. Chemical
    C. Cellular
    D. Extrinsic

91. The American Cancer Society recommends which skin cancer prevention guideline?

    A. Avoid direct sun exposure from 9 a.m. to 3 p.m.
    B. Wear clothing that covers the skin and a hat with a wide brim
    C. Use tanning booths and sun lamps no more than twice weekly
    D. Apply sunscreen with a sun protection factor (SPF) of 15 or greater

92. Which microorganism is associated with liver cancer?

    A. *Helicobacter pylori*
    B. Epstein-Barr virus (EBV)
    C. HIV type 1 (HIV-1)
    D. Hepatitis B virus (HBV)

93. A patient receiving treatment for cancer expresses concern regarding the impact the illness will have on their career. What statement could the nurse include in the discussion with the patient?

    A. "There are no legal protections for people who want to return to work after cancer treatment."
    B. "Don't worry about your job until you're further into your recovery."
    C. "You could always apply for another job."
    D. "Most cancer survivors do return to work."

94. An oncology nurse is coordinating a prostate screening event at a health fair. Participants will be able to receive a blood test for the prostate-specific antigen and a digital exam from a healthcare provider. This event is focused on which level of prevention?

    A. Primary
    B. Secondary
    C. Tertiary
    D. Quaternary

95. Which rehabilitation measures for survivors reduce symptom burden and emphasize comfort?

    A. Preventive
    B. Restorative
    C. Supportive
    D. Palliative

96. Which age group of cancer survivors is more likely to be uninsured or underinsured?

    A. 15 to 39 years
    B. Birth to 5 years
    C. 40 to 64 years
    D. 65 years and older

97. The care team is developing a care plan for a patient diagnosed with breast cancer. The treatment plan includes mastectomy and chemotherapy. What intervention will the team consider to provide supportive rehabilitation?

    A. Educating the patient about prosthetic bras
    B. Providing ice therapy for the prevention of hair loss
    C. Developing a program to return the patient to pre-diagnosis activity level
    D. Administering antiemetics to prevent nausea and vomiting

98. A young adult patient who is diagnosed with sarcoma and is a former marathon runner completes cancer treatment. The patient begins training to compete again. This type of rehabilitation is:

    A. Preventive
    B. Restorative
    C. Supportive
    D. Palliative

99. During a follow-up clinic appointment, a 20-year-old survivor of leukemia seems especially concerned that a close friend has been diagnosed with cancer. Before sending the patient for routine blood work, the nurse takes a few minutes to find out more about the patient's concerns, which are likely related to anxiety regarding:

   A. Fatigue
   B. Rejection
   C. Recurrence
   D. Treatment decisions

100. During a breast cancer patient's posttreatment visit, the oncology nurse uses which assessment tool when the patient expresses a fear of recurrence?

   A. CINV (chemotherapy-induced nausea and vomiting) grading scale
   B. Mucositis grading scale
   C. Distress thermometer rating scale
   D. Pain diary record

101. An oncology nurse plans counseling topics for a small group of adolescent patients diagnosed with cancer and their parents in preparation for treatment. Sexual health content should include:

   A. Exclusively information on anatomy
   B. Importance of abstinence until treatment completion
   C. Minimal information because the parents will discuss more information with the patient
   D. Safe sex information and possible late physical effects of treatment on reproductive systems

102. For cancer survivors, anxiety, depression, and fear of recurrence are part of which type of nursing assessment?

   A. Prevention
   B. Physical
   C. Mobility
   D. Psychosocial

103. The definition of cancer survivor applies:

    A. Only to patients who have survived for 5 or more years after starting treatment

    B. As soon as treatment has been deemed successful

    C. To any patient diagnosed with cancer throughout the rest of their lifetime

    D. Specifically to patients who had childhood cancer and survived to adulthood

104. Which types of support referrals should the nurse make for a patient who expresses loss of libido, erectile dysfunction, and inability to be intimate with a partner?

    A. A counselor to discuss any psychologic issues

    B. A counselor to discuss sexual and social concerns and a primary provider/oncologist to assess physical issues

    C. A primary oncologist to assess any physical issues

    D. No referral, because these symptoms are typical after treatment, and the patient just needs time to adjust

105. The palliative care oncology nurse may administer ondansetron (Zofran) in order to treat which potential end-of-life symptom?

    A. Nausea

    B. Constipation

    C. Pain

    D. Delirium

106. A legal document that details a patient's preferences for healthcare and end-of-life care is known as a:

    A. POLST

    B. Power of attorney

    C. Advance directive

    D. DNR

107. The nurse knows to assess for which common side effect associated with nonsteroidal anti-inflammatory drugs (NSAIDs)?

    A. Neutropenia
    B. Rash
    C. Dyspepsia
    D. Headache

108. The oncology patient scores a 7 on the National Comprehensive Cancer Network (NCCN) distress thermometer. What is the most appropriate next step for the nurse to take?

    A. Provide antidepressant medication to the patient
    B. Refer the patient for further evaluation and psychosocial services
    C. Reevaluate the patient's score in 1 week
    D. Document the score in the patient's chart

109. The nurse is caring for a hospice patient with dysphagia who is having difficulty swallowing pills. The nurse intervenes by:

    A. Crushing all of the patient's medications and mixing them with applesauce for easier swallowing
    B. Referring the patient to speech therapy to improve the dysphagia
    C. Evaluating the need for each medication and working with the provider to simplify the regimen
    D. Educating the patient on the importance of medication adherence

110. Which drug is preferred for managing end-of-life seizures in the oncology patient?

    A. Gabapentin
    B. Lorazepam
    C. Levetiracetam
    D. Morphine

111. The nurse is performing a spiritual assessment on a patient with advanced cancer. What should be included?

    A. Patient's religious/spiritual background, beliefs, and preferred practices
    B. Nurse's own beliefs religious and spiritual beliefs
    C. Nothing; a spiritual assessment is not indicated
    D. Patient's socioeconomic status

112. The nurse is speaking to a patient with advanced lung cancer. What should be considered in discussing advanced cancer and end-of-life issues?

    A. That hospice services only take place at home

    B. The patient's cultural and religious beliefs and norms

    C. The patient's insurance type

    D. The availability of clinical trials

113. The oncology nurse is educating a patient with prostate cancer on the potential side effects of leuprorelin. Which information should the nurse include?

    A. Libido is likely to increase while on endocrine therapy

    B. Fertility should remain normal

    C. Breasts may become enlarged from this type of therapy

    D. This medication may cause hirsutism

114. A patient diagnosed with breast cancer 4 years ago refused all treatment, and the cancer has now progressed into a large, fungating wound on the breast. Upon assessment, it is discovered that the patient may have refused treatment based on culturally related medical practices. What question will best assist the nurse in addressing the primary need in this patent?

    A. "What cultural practices did you engage in when you were first diagnosed with breast cancer?"

    B. "How do you feel the healthcare team can best help you through the next stage of your cancer treatment?"

    C. "What herbs and supplements do you include in your current therapy regimen?"

    D. "Are there certain cultural or spiritual practices we can facilitate for you during your treatment?"

115. Which patient would cause the nurse the most concern regarding the development of sexual intimacy issues?

    A. 25-year-old patient with curative intent testicular cancer

    B. 45-year-old patient with terminal lung cancer

    C. 42-year-old patient with curative intent breast cancer

    D. 33-year-old patient with basal cell carcinoma of the skin

116. A 27-year-old patient who was assigned female at birth is preparing to start a new chemotherapy regimen. Which referral should the nurse prioritize?

    A. Reproductive medicine
    B. Psychiatry
    C. Pain management
    D. Free wig program

117. The accumulation of lymph fluid in interstitial spaces is known by what term?

    A. Lymphadenopathy
    B. Lymphoma
    C. Lymphedema
    D. Endolymph

118. Which model is used to discuss sexuality and intimacy issues with patients?

    A. CAGE
    B. PLISSIT
    C. ADPIE
    D. Motivational interviewing

119. A patient presents with symptomatic hypothyroidism 9 months after completing radiation for tonsil cancer. The nurse refers to the patient's hypothyroidism as a(n):

    A. Long-term side effect
    B. Acute side effect
    C. Late effect
    D. Unrelated effect

120. Which factor presents the highest risk for fatigue during cancer treatment?

    A. Single-agent chemotherapy
    B. Obesity
    C. Smoking
    D. Opioid use

121. The nurse has provided a patient with strategies for improving lymphedema. The nurse will provide clarification if the patient indicates they will use what measure?

    A. Elevating the affected extremity

    B. Maintaining a healthy weight

    C. Avoiding prolonged standing

    D. Applying heat packs to the affected area

122. What age group is at the highest risk for altered body image related to disease and treatment changes?

    A. Children

    B. Young adults

    C. Middle-aged adults

    D. Older adults

123. The nurse prepares the patient for the expected timeline of chemotherapy-induced alopecia by stating:

    A. "Hair loss will typically begin within a day after starting chemotherapy; your hair will start to regrow as soon as you receive your last dose."

    B. "Hair loss will typically begin 2 weeks after you start chemotherapy; your hair will start to regrow 6 to 8 weeks after you receive your last dose."

    C. "Hair loss typically starts a month after you start chemotherapy; your hair will likely not regrow after you complete chemotherapy."

    D. "Hair loss will typically occur on your head only; you will not lose body hair."

124. What comorbidity is a contraindication to an orthoptic neobladder creation?

    A. History of nephrolithiasis

    B. Irritable bowel disease

    C. Recurrent urinary tract infections

    D. Herpes simplex virus

125. What patient should the nurse advise against taking nonsteroidal anti-inflammatory drugs (NSAIDs)?

    A. 45-year-old patient with cirrhosis
    B. 68-year-old patient with renal insufficiency
    C. 36-year-old patient with migraines
    D. 64-year-old patient with breast cancer

126. Which temperature is considered the threshold for fever in neutropenic patients and warrants antibiotics?

    A. Single oral temperature of 100.4°F
    B. Single oral temperature of 101°F
    C. Oral temperature of 101°F sustained over 1 hour
    D. Single rectal temperature of 101°F

127. A patient reports running out of oxycodone 2 days ago and presents to the clinic visibly diaphoretic, anxious, and vomiting. What is the nurse most concerned about?

    A. Opioid addiction
    B. Panic attack
    C. Medication allergy
    D. Opioid withdrawal

128. A patient with lung cancer is prescribed sertraline (Zoloft) for depression. When educating the patient, which is an important point to include?

    A. It is all right to stop the medication whenever you begin to feel better
    B. It can take 2 to 4 weeks for the medication to start having an effect
    C. This medication typically causes somnolence
    D. You should not drive while on this medication

129. Which type of therapy is an example of a mind–body intervention?

    A. Tai chi
    B. Biofield therapy
    C. Chiropractic therapy
    D. Meditation

130. Tai chi is an example of:

    A. Exercise therapy

    B. Manipulative therapy

    C. Mind–body intervention

    D. Energy therapy

131. A patient on nivolumab asks the nurse about using herbal supplements to help boost the immune system. Which is the nurse's best response?

    A. "Herbal supplements are natural and therefore are safe to take while you are receiving treatment."

    B. "While many herbal supplements are safe, we do not yet know how they interact with nivolumab."

    C. "You will need to see a herbalist because we do not discuss supplements in the oncology office."

    D. "You should make sure to take the herbal supplements only on days you are not receiving treatment."

132. The National Center for Complementary and Integrative Health (NCCIH) categorizes complementary health techniques into which two subgroups?

    A. Evidence-based and theoretical

    B. Approved and experimental

    C. Natural products and mind–body practices

    D. Safe and risky

133. When should palliative care begin?

    A. At initial cancer diagnosis

    B. At progression of the disease

    C. When life expectancy is 6 months or less

    D. When pain first develops

134. A patient expresses interest in undergoing acupuncture as a complementary therapy for cancer. Which lab results are most important for the nurse to review?

    A. Complete blood count (CBC) with differential

    B. Basic metabolic panel (BMP)

    C. Liver enzymes

    D. Thyroid panel

135. Which is the primary location for hematopoiesis in adults?

    A. Bone marrow

    B. Spleen

    C. Lymph nodes

    D. Liver

136. The nurse knows that the patient requires further education about eligibility for Medicare-based hospice care when they state:

    A. "I will need have two physicians estimate a life expectancy of 6 months or less."

    B. "I will need to be eligible for Medicare Part A first."

    C. "I will need consent to hospice care before I can receive it."

    D. "I will need to forgo all doctor visits to be eligible."

137. A patient is receiving granulocyte colony-stimulating factor (G-CSF) following chemotherapy. What does the nurse include in the patient's education?

    A. You may experience bone pain with this medication

    B. You do not need to follow neutropenic precautions after receiving this medication

    C. Fever is a possible side effect of this medication

    D. This medication is given only after your labs show you are neutropenic

138. Which absolute neutrophil count (ANC) is considered a grade 3 neutropenia?

    A. $1,800/mm^3$

    B. $1,600/mm^3$

    C. $880/mm^3$

    D. $490/mm^3$

139. A benefit of radiation therapy as compared with chemotherapy is:

    A. Radiation therapy requires less pretreatment planning than chemotherapy

    B. Radiation therapy kills tumor cells and minimizes damage to other organs

    C. Radiation therapy does not require multiple providers to be involved in the patient's treatment

    D. Radiation therapy is always covered by insurance

140. A patient who received carboplatin and docetaxel 10 days ago presents with chills, malaise, and dysuria. Which is the nurse's best next step?

   A. Check urinalysis (UA)
   B. Check complete blood count (CBC) with differential
   C. Auscultate the patient's lungs
   D. Auscultate the patient's bowel sounds

141. What is the purpose of radiation simulation?

   A. To get the patient oriented to the radiation treatment process
   B. To ensure the patient can lie still for the duration of treatment
   C. To determine the radiation treatment and target volume
   D. To assess the tumor's sensitivity to ionizing radiation

142. Ionizing radiation is most effective on cells during which phase?

   A. Growth
   B. DNA synthesis
   C. Mitosis
   D. Rest

143. Which mode of treatment involves radiation being delivered in or near the tumor?

   A. Brachytherapy
   B. Intensity-modulated radiation therapy
   C. Stereotactic radiosurgery
   D. Proton beam therapy

144. Which radiation dose equation is correct?

   A. 1 Gy = 100 rad
   B. 1 rad = 10 cGy
   C. 1 Gy = 10 rad
   D. 1 cGy = 20 rad

145. A patient who completed radiation for oropharyngeal carcinoma 1 year ago returns for follow-up and asks the nurse why they need to have blood work performed. The nurse educates the patient by responding:

    A. "Radiation to the head and neck can cause delayed hypothyroidism."
    B. "The radiation oncology team assumes responsibility for annual blood work."
    C. "Radiation therapy can increase your risk of hyperlipidemia."
    D. "Your blood work results can help identify disease recurrence."

146. A patient planned for proton therapy inquires about the benefit of receiving proton therapy as opposed to traditional radiation therapy. The nurse's best response is:

    A. "You will need fewer sessions of proton therapy."
    B. "Proton therapy can be used with a broader range of cancer types."
    C. "Proton therapy is offered at more facilities, so it is more convenient for you."
    D. "Proton therapy will likely cause less damage to surrounding tissue."

147. A patient who received radiation to the tonsils 6 months ago presents for follow-up. During the nursing assessment, the patient reports fatigue and unexplained weight gain. Which question should the nurse ask to further evaluate the potential etiology?

    A. "Do you have trouble breathing when you walk?"
    B. "Have you noticed brittle hair and nails or intolerance to cold?"
    C. "Do you have a rash in the area of the previous radiation?"
    D. "Do you feel depressed?"

148. An older adult patient with a 30-year history of cigarette smoking presents to the clinic during week 3 of radiation treatment to the right breast. In assessing the patient for toxicities, what body system should the nurse prioritize?

    A. Integumentary
    B. Cardiovascular
    C. Digestive
    D. Immune

149. Which serum sodium range would be considered moderate hyponatremia?

    A. 140 to 145 mmol/L

    B. 130 to 134 mmol/L

    C. 125 to 129 mmol/L

    D. 115 to 120 mmol/L

150. A patient with disseminated intravascular coagulation (DIC) has been stabilized for discharge from the hospital. The nurse's discharge education should include which important safety point?

    A. Avoid contact with fresh flowers in soil

    B. Avoid nonsteroidal anti-inflammatory drugs (NSAIDs)

    C. Engage in a daily weight-lifting activity to gain strength

    D. Maintain a low-fat, high-protein diet

151. The nurse is caring for a patient with sepsis and reviews the provider's orders to administer intravenous vancomycin and obtain sputum and blood cultures. Which statement is true?

    A. Sputum and blood cultures should be obtained before starting the vancomycin

    B. The vancomycin should be started first as this is most important to treat the infection

    C. One set of blood cultures is sufficient when evaluating for sepsis

    D. Sputum culture is not necessary unless the patient is experiencing dyspnea

152. The most common pathogenic causes of sepsis in the United States are:

    A. Fungal infections

    B. Viral infections

    C. Gram-positive bacterial infections

    D. Gram-negative bacterial infections

153. A 22-year-old patient reports switching from cigarettes to chewing tobacco to "be healthier." The nurse prioritizes:

    A. Discussing that chewing tobacco and cigarettes both cause lung cancer

    B. Applauding the patient for finding a healthier alternative to cigarettes

    C. Providing patient education on esophageal and oral cancers

    D. Referring the patient to a lung cancer screening program

154. The nurse is assessing a patient's vital signs and finds the following: temperature of 101.4°F, blood pressure of 80/50, heart rate of 132 beats/min, and pulse oximetry of 87%. Which is the most appropriate next step?

    A. Administering acetaminophen
    B. Performing an EKG
    C. Drawing labs
    D. Placing the patient on oxygen

155. Which pattern of cancer risk is accurate?

    A. Cancer incidence is higher above age 55 years
    B. Cancer incidence peaks between ages 30 and 50 years
    C. Cancer incidence is highest in childhood and then again after age 60 years
    D. Cancer risk affects all ages equally

156. Which patient group has the highest incidence rate of cervical cancer?

    A. Hispanic/Latinx patients
    B. Asian patients
    C. African American patients
    D. White patients

157. A patient who received radiation 6 months ago for oropharyngeal cancer reports chronic xerostomia. The nurse includes which important teaching point?

    A. Maintain good oral hygiene with regular dental visits
    B. Eat acidic foods often
    C. Rinse with hydrogen peroxide daily
    D. Avoid fluoride-containing toothpastes

158. A nurse is organizing a prostate cancer screening event in the community, and knows to focus outreach on which higher-risk population?

    A. Asian patients
    B. White patients
    C. African American patients
    D. Hispanic/Latinx patients

159. A patient who recently received radiation to the right breast informs the nurse they will be taking an airplane soon to go on vacation. The nurse prioritizes which teaching point?

   A. Avoid carrying luggage with your left arm
   B. Wear a compression sleeve on your right arm while flying
   C. Take prophylactic antibiotics during the trip
   D. Avoid submerging the right breast in water

160. A patient reports dysphagia since completing chemoradiation treatment. During the nurse's assessment, the patient is noted to have dyspnea and a productive cough. Which is the next step the nurse will take?

   A. Administer guaifenesin as needed
   B. Refer the patient to speech therapy
   C. Auscultate the patient's lungs
   D. Encourage the patient to continue eating to improve the dysphagia

161. What is the most common histopathologic breast cancer classification?

   A. Ductal adenocarcinoma
   B. Lobular carcinoma
   C. Papillary carcinoma
   D. Inflammatory carcinoma

162. Endocrine therapy is most likely to lead to a favorable prognosis in which type of breast cancer?

   A. Luminal A tumors
   B. Luminal B tumors
   C. Normal-like breast tumors
   D. Basal tumors

163. A patient newly diagnosed with breast cancer, classified as grade 1 on the Bloom–Richardson grading system, inquires as to what this means. The nurse responds that grade 1 indicates that:

   A. The tumor is well differentiated—the tumor cells look similar to those of the original tissue
   B. The tumor is poorly differentiated—the tumor cells look very different from those of the original tissue
   C. No metastasis has occurred yet
   D. The cancer is present only in one lymph node

164. Which molecular classification applies to oropharyngeal carcinomas?

   A. Epstein-Barr virus (EBV)
   B. Human papillomavirus (HPV)
   C. Human epidermal growth factor receptor 2 (HER2)
   D. Epidermal growth factor receptor (EGFR)

165. What do T, N, and M stand for in a cancer diagnosis?

   A. Type, nodes, metastases
   B. Tumor, necrosis, mutations
   C. Tumor, nodes, metastases
   D. Tumor necrosis, nodes, mitosis

Practice Exam Answers With Rationales

1. A) Villous
Among villous, tubular, and tubulovillous histologies, villous adenomas are at highest risk of becoming malignant. Multiploid is not a histologic type.

2. C) Adenocarcinoma
Adenocarcinomas make up about 95% of colorectal cancers. Carcinoid, squamous, and lymphoid are far less common histologic types of colorectal cancer.

3. A) Helps the patient access healthcare and overcome barriers in the system
The main role of the ONN is to improve patients' access to oncology care, not to recruit patients to sites. The ONN serves all patients with cancer, not just those with high needs. ONNs do not act as social workers.

4. A) Oncology Nursing Society (ONS)
ONS is responsible for establishing standards for the practice of oncology nursing. ANA represents nurses in the United States more broadly. TJC accredits U.S. healthcare establishments. ANCC is responsible for certifying advanced practice nurses.

5. A) Nursing interventions documented at the end of shift
Quality nursing documentation should ideally be noted in real time as events transpire rather than all at once at the end of the shift. Documenting changes in the patient's condition, documenting events and interventions in sequential order, and including objective nursing judgment in documentation all reflect proper, quality documentation.

6. D) Select states regardless of where they obtained their nursing license
The nursing licensure compact allows nurses to practice in select states (currently about 30 states participate) other than the one in which they obtained their license without needing to obtain a new license. It does not apply to all states, and there is no grace period involved. The compact does not affect a nurse's ability to work in multiple hospitals.

7. B) PRoQOL

PRoQOL, or the Professional Quality of Life Scale, is the most used tool for evaluating compassion fatigue. PLISSIT (Permission, Limited Information, Specific Suggestions, Intensive Therapy) is a model used for discussing sexual concerns with patients. CAGE is a mnemonic for an assessment questionnaire for alcohol use. ABC refers to prioritization of airway, breathing, and circulation.

8. D) To provide accreditation to healthcare organizations

The role of The Joint Commission is to verify that healthcare organizations are practicing according to a standard of care and to provide accreditation accordingly. The Joint Commission is not specifically tasked with overseeing nursing procedures. It is also not responsible for malpractice investigations or developing nursing education standards.

9. B) Autonomy

Autonomy refers to an individual's right to self-determination. The equitable allocation of healthcare resources is the essence of justice. Beneficence is the act of doing good, while nonmaleficence is the basic duty to avoid harming patients.

10. C) Consumer advocacy

Consumer advocacy refers to the nurse's role in providing adequate information to the patient. The nurse's responsibility to represent the patient's best interests is called simplistic advocacy. A nurse practicing paternalistic advocacy is taking an action they believe is beneficial to their patient without first securing their patient's consent. Existential advocacy refers to a nurse's duty to accept and support a patient's beliefs and values.

11. A) It instills confidence in the public that the nurse has the proper education and training

The main benefit of oncology nursing certification is that it increases the public's confidence that an oncology nurse has a thorough education and adequate training. While it may also instill self-confidence in the nurse, that is not the main objective. Oncology nursing certification does not aim to justify wages or assess nursing education deficits.

12. C) Assess for psychiatric disorders or coexisting pain

When a patient expresses a wish to die, it is a priority for the nurse to ensure that the patient does not have a psychiatric condition or uncontrolled pain that is influencing those feelings. Editing the advance directive may be indicated if the patient wishes to add a do-not-resuscitate (DNR) order, but the directives are not related to euthanasia. It is inappropriate to reinforce the notion that life is worth living or to refer the patient to another state for further care.

13. A) Practice to the full extent of their education

The duties of taking vital signs and assisting patients to the bathroom are aspects of patient care, but they do not reflect working to a nurse's full potential with regard to education and training. The IOM report does not state that nurses should participate in all aspects of patient care, nor does it recommend a minimum academic degree. The duties described do not contradict the recommendation to involve nurses in policy development.

14. C) 1,000 hours within the past 2.5 years

A prerequisite to becoming an OCN is the completion of a minimum of 1,000 practice hours in oncology within the 2.5 years prior to applying.

15. D) Systematic review of randomized clinical trials

A systematic review of randomized clinical trials is considered the strongest category of research-based evidence, followed by a randomized clinical trial at a single site. Case studies and systematic reviews of qualitative studies may be helpful but are considered to be weaker types of evidence.

16. D) Single-site qualitative study

A systematic review of randomized clinical trials is considered the strongest type of evidence. Cohort studies provide a moderate degree of evidence strength. Systematic reviews of qualitative studies are more impactful than a single-site qualitative study.

17. C) 5%

Severe hypersensitivity reactions are rare. The overall incidence rate of severe reactions is approximately 5%.

18. A) SPIKES
SPIKES is a communication tool used in palliative and end-of-life decision-making. SPIKES stands for setting, perception, invitation, knowledge, emotions, strategy/summary. FACES is a mnemonic device for pain measurement. MMSE stands for Mini Mental State Examination. PQRST is used to assess pain.

19. B) Hypotension
Taxanes are chemotherapy agents known to have a high incidence of hypersensitivity. These signs include anaphylaxis, facial flushing, and hypotension. Atrial fibrillation, incontinence, and ataxia are not signs of hypersensitivity in taxane agents.

20. B) Asparaginases
Asparaginases, taxanes, platinum salts, and monoclonal antibodies have the highest potential for hypersensitivity reactions. Anthracyclines like doxorubicin and dacarbazines like methotrexate have occasional potential. Antimetabolites like hydroxyurea have rare potential.

21. B) Hypercalcemia
Hypercalcemia causes fatigue and muscle spasms. The patient also becomes hypertensive and bradycardic. A central line infection would cause fever, chills, pain, redness, and swelling at the central line site. Urinary tract infections cause frequent urination with pain or burning. Bowel obstruction causes abdominal pain and swelling, loss of appetite, and vomiting.

22. B) Anaphylaxis
Monoclonal antibodies can trigger anaphylaxis with a rapid onset of symptoms like anxiety and breathing difficulties. Monoclonal antibodies can cause hypotension, not hypertension. They are not known to cause rhabdomyolysis or malignant hyperthermia.

23. A) 10 or more years after radiation treatment
Radiation-associated solid tumors are common secondary malignancies. They usually appear 10 or more years after a pediatric patient has received treatment.

24. C) 10% to 30%
Hypercalcemia occurs in 10% to 30% of cancer patients over the course of their disease process and presents most frequently in breast cancer, squamous cell lung cancer, and multiple myeloma.

25. C) Takes into account cultural characteristics that may affect the key caregiver's role
The nurse knows to identify the key caregiver and recognize that caregiving roles vary between families and cultures. The nurse will teach all caregivers proper patient care, not just the key caregiver. It would be irresponsible for the nurse to rely on one caregiver to train another. The patient or legally appointed representative should identify the key caregiver, and there is no need to restrict selection by gender or relationship unless that is the patient's wish.

26. B) Cleaning and dressing the patient's body
After the patient's death, the nurse will prepare the body to appear as natural as possible and remove tubes and equipment to help the family develop a less painful memory of the loved one. The nurse will allow the family to be present at the moment of death and follow the family's wishes as to the removal of the patient's body.

27. C) Hydromorphone is a rapid-release analgesic, and transdermal fentanyl is a long-acting analgesic
Patients experiencing breakthrough pain need a rapid-release analgesic such as hydromorphone and a long-acting analgesic such as transdermal fentanyl. Hydromorphone is not stronger than fentanyl, nor does transdermal fentanyl need hydromorphone to be effective.

28. B) Chaplain
Interdisciplinary hospice teams include volunteers, chaplains, oncologists, and nurses, many of whom will be available to address the patient's needs. In the case of spiritual distress, the chaplain will be the team member best suited to address the patient's spiritual needs.

29. B) They should follow up with the patient within 24 to 48 hours after the patient returns home

The nurse will call the patient within 24 to 48 hours of the patient's returning home after treatment to ensure that the patient is following antiemetic measures. Emetogenic treatments can cause serious, severe, life-threatening nausea and vomiting. The patient is not safe to drive and may develop hypovolemia from vomiting, not hypervolemia.

30. B) Are most often used with pharmacologic methods to relieve pain

Nonpharmacologic methods such as acupuncture, massage, and guided imagery are most often used with pharmacologic methods to relieve pain. Studies show that nonpharmacologic methods are useful as adjuncts to pharmacologic methods but typically are not sufficient alone for pain control. Nonpharmacologic methods do not last longer than pharmacologic methods. There is no evidence that non-pharmacologic methods should not be used for severe pain.

31. B) Liver

The liver is the primary site of metastasis. Approximately 20% of colorectal cancer patients have synchronous liver metastases. About 70% of patients not cured of colorectal cancer will develop liver metastases. Colorectal cancer that invades the vascular system can also spread to the brain, bones, kidneys, and adrenal glands. Lung metastasis is rare. The spleen and stomach are not common sites of metastasis.

32. C) Followed up with radical inguinal orchiectomy

Suspicious testicular masses should be followed up with a radical inguinal orchiectomy for diagnosis, not biopsied in situ, monitored for 3 months, or examined with a scan such as CT. Radical inguinal orchiectomy removes the primary cancer site from the body immediately to prevent metastasis.

33. A) Encourage slowly acknowledging and including changes into daily activities and social relationships

When providing care for a young adult patient with altered body image, the most appropriate step would be to encourage the patient to slowly acknowledge how their body has changed and why, then make a plan to integrate this into daily living and relationships. Providing resources and educating on self-affirming statements are options that may be helpful but are not the most appropriate because these interventions do not address the altered body image when in social settings. Allowing the patient to express concerns is a caring approach; however, offering false hope is not appropriate.

34. C) Kinesthetic
Kinesthetic learners retain concepts and information best by doing and therefore would benefit from being allowed to demonstrate what they have learned. Visual learners learn by watching. Global learners need the overall big picture to help map concepts, while analytical learners need things broken down into smaller chunks of information.

35. A) Denial
The patient is exhibiting signs of denial that include the rejection of real situations and associated feelings. Suppression is the conscious refusal to acknowledge a difficult situation. Displacement is the transferring of emotions from person or object to another, less-threatening one. Rationalization involves justifying illogical ideas or feelings by using acceptable explanations.

36. B) Conduct a needs and abilities assessment of the patient's family and caregiver
The first step to address the patient's concerns is to conduct an assessment of the family and caregiver to determine if their needs are being met and if they have the ability to provide long-term care. Illness has an impact on the entire family, and the nurse is responsible for ensuring caregivers have the tools needed to understand the impact as well as care for the patient. Referring the patient for psychosocial counseling and counseling on nutrition and food choices may be helpful but does not address the patient's worry about the caregiver relationship. Ordering corticosteroid medications may be helpful in addressing the alopecia but does not address the primary concern.

37. D) Ensuring that patient beliefs are accepted and supported
Existential advocacy is the interaction of nurse and patient that allows for an understanding of how the patient experiences health, illness, suffering, or dying. Ensuring that a patient's beliefs are accepted and supported is an example of this type of advocacy. Providing information and supporting decisions is an example of consumer-centric advocacy. Ensuring patients have adequate, accurate information is an example of consumer advocacy. Doing something on behalf of the patient for their own good is an example of paternalistic advocacy.

38. C) Assess the patient's stress and coping mechanisms
The primary need in this patient is to address the inability to effectively cope with stress and the diagnosis. Therefore, the first step is to assess the patient's stress, stressors, and coping mechanisms to make an accurate and complete nursing care plan. Providing support for the family and friends is not a primary need for the patient. Educating the patient and family on coping skills would be conducted after the assessment. Admitting the patient to an inpatient rehabilitation facility is not indicated at this point.

39. B) Assess the family as a whole and the ability to collectively care for the patient
Assessing the family as a whole to determine the ability of the group to collectively care for the patient and assigning primary and secondary caregiver roles as needed will be the nurse's first action. Referring the family to counseling and support would not be the first step to take to determine the family's ability to care for the patient. A list of community resources may be needed for the patient and the family but is not the first step. Admission to a palliative care facility would be reserved for when the patient cannot be at home and would not be a first step to address the patient's need.

40. B) Refer the patient to a support group for breast cancer survivors
Referring the patient to a support group that is focused on the experiences of similar patients is the best option when a patient is making critical decisions about care and is concerned about effects and outcomes. Providing information on breast reconstruction is appropriate but is not the best way to address the underlying cause of the patient's concerns. Scheduling a consultation with a plastic surgeon is premature and would not be the best step to take at this time. Encouraging the patient to seek counsel may be appropriate for some patients, but not all, and therefore would not be the best way to address the concerns of the patient.

41. C) Anticipatory
When a patient and family members have experienced a long battle with a disease, there is a tendency to go through anticipatory grief in preparation for death, which may often be inevitable. This form of grief is experienced during the patient's life and throughout the active disease process. Inhibited grief is a form of grief that is suppressed. Delayed grief involves intentionally suppressing grief until another time that is more conducive to the grieving process. Disenfranchised grief is seen in people who are unable to acknowledge the grief of others.

42. A) Exacerbating pain

Complications from the progression of disease such as anxiety and fatigue can impact the patient in negative ways, such as by exacerbating pain. Many medications used to treat disease symptoms will cause constipation, but not anxiety. Anxiety does not directly cause an increase in caregiver burden or a risk for drug misuse. There are other impacting factors that contribute to caregiver burden and drug misuse.

43. C) Refer for psychiatric admission and evaluation

The priority intervention for this patient would be to refer for psychiatric evaluation as the patient has expressed a tendency toward suicidal ideation. Contacting the provider will be necessary, but not for adjusting the dosage for treatment or for prescribing corticosteroids. This may be a decision that comes later, but it is not a priority intervention. Referral to a nutritionist may be an intervention that is needed once the patient is stabilized by the psychiatric provider.

44. B) Encourage the patient to discuss feelings

At the first signs of depression, the nurse will encourage the patient to discuss their feelings to build a trusting relationship and evaluate for severity of psychologic effects. Referring the patient for psychiatric evaluation and reporting to the provider are not indicated right away because the nurse would first perform an assessment. Reassuring the patient is never a good practice as it could be interpreted as an uncaring diversion to avoid the issue at hand.

45. A) Postoperative care and support

The patient lives alone and is undergoing a very challenging and aggressive surgery that will require support and care after discharge from the hospital. Ensuring the patient has the appropriate caregiver and support system is critical. While providing information on fertility preservation may be important, the patient has already made this decision and most likely has had eggs extracted in preparation for surgery. Counseling for altered body image may be needed, but this will be discussed as the patient heals. Access to community services and supplies would be a focus should the patient be homebound with no access to support.

46. D) Optimism and motivation are decreased, which impedes the patient's ability to meet treatment goals

A loss of personal control is a perception that one's own abilities or activities will not be sufficient to control their situation. Therefore, optimism and motivation levels will be lower and may impact the overall treatment goals. Self-efficacy is the perceived ability to cope in certain situations; however, when self-efficacy is affected, it does not mean the patient will not adhere to treatment plans. Adjusting to the disease is facilitated by a patient's beliefs and desires, not their emotional response. The emotional response would be the adjustment to the disease. Feelings of anxiety and stress are not replaced and may still be viable feelings in a patient with loss of personal control.

47. B) Alleviation of bothersome symptoms

Palliation in the context of patient care refers to symptom management. As such, it is a component of all patient care. While patients receiving palliative care may require large doses of opioids, palliation is not limited to pharmacologic pain management. The decision to forego life-saving treatments can be a component of palliation but only if it helps alleviate symptoms. Palliation is not dependent on expected survival.

48. B) Methylnaltrexone (Relistor) injection, 8 mg subcutaneously every other day for 10 days

Methylnaltrexone is a peripherally acting opioid antagonist that inhibits the delayed gastric motility and reduced transit associated with opioids. Methylcellulose, a bulk-forming laxative, is not appropriate for older adults who may not adequately hydrate to move the laxative through the gastrointestinal tract. Naltrexone is an opioid antagonist but is not indicated for opioid-induced constipation. IM naltrexone administration would induce acute opioid withdrawal in the patient. Naloxone is also an opioid antagonist, but its primary use is as treatment of opioid intoxication and associated respiratory depression.

49. C) Adjuvant, nonpharmacologic comfort measures

Nonpharmacologic, adjuvant comfort measures such as transcutaneous electrical nerve stimulation (TENS) therapy, guided imagery, music, and massage can help patients control breakthrough pain in conjunction with pharmacologic measures. When a patient is experiencing pain, it is not an appropriate time to suggest focusing on life review, putting affairs in order, or having visits with family and friends.

50. A) The patient begins pulling at the IV tubing. Agitation continues 30 minutes after alprazolam 1 mg IV is given, so the nurse contacts the ordering provider for additional options

The principle of double effect holds that a provider's actions are justified, even if an adverse outcome is possible, so long as the intent is for a good outcome and no other option is available with a lesser risk of a bad outcome. Administering IV alprazolam as ordered to an agitated patient could cause central nervous system depression; however the intent implied is alleviation of agitation and reduced risk of harm to self. If a patient cannot verbally communicate troubling symptoms, the nurse must assess nonverbal cues. It is inappropriate for the nurse to treat a patient's condition based on personal convictions. Nursing judgment is not a substitution for an order. While gasping respirations may indicate an air-hungry patient, the implied intent of morphine administration is to reduce the nuisance to the patient's roommate.

51. B) Papilledema

Papilledema is considered cardinal sign of ICP. Brain metastases is a risk factor for ICP. Headaches can be an early or late symptom of ICP. Peripheral edema is not associated with ICP.

52. C) Nurses report a lack of time and knowledge to help patients with advance directives

Nurses typically report that they do not have enough time or knowledge of the topic to help patients with advance directives. An advance directive aids patient autonomy by allowing the patient to document their wishes for healthcare so that these wishes can be carried out when the patient is no longer able to personally communicate them. Nursing care includes advocating for patient autonomy, so the nurse bears a responsibility to speak to the patient and family about advance directives. Patients with advance directives are more likely to receive their chosen end-of-life care.

53. B) Pain

More than 95% of patients with SCC have pain. Tachycardia and Horner syndrome occur with superior vena cava syndrome. Rash is a side effect of some chemotherapy treatments, but it is not a symptoms of SCC.

54. B) Increased intracranial pressure

An Ommaya reservoir is a port in the intracranial space used for treatment. Headaches, nausea, vomiting, and weakness are all early signs of increased intracranial pressure. Anaphylaxis, superior vena cava syndrome, and spinal cord compression do not have this combination of symptoms.

55. C) Lung cancer
Right-sided lung cancers are responsible for most cases of SVCS. The superior vena cava is in the mediastinum. The mediastinum also contains the right bronchus to the lung. Patients with small cell and non-small cell lung cancers are most often at risk for SVCS. Breast cancer tumors and sarcomas could have potential malignancies that cause SVCS, but not as often as lung cancers.

56. C) Superior vena cava syndrome (SVCS)
Swelling of the neck and face and distended veins are signs of SVCS. These are not signs of anaphylaxis, which usually presents as shortness of breath and itching. ICP is marked by headache, nausea and vomiting, and weakness. SCC symptoms include pain, weakness, and sensory loss.

57. C) Put the patient on bed rest and elevate head of bed 30 degrees
Patients with Ommaya reservoirs are at higher risk for developing increased intracranial pressure (ICP) due to occlusion of reservoir lines. A patient with an Ommaya reservoir who exhibits these symptoms should be positioned with head of the bed at 30 degrees, and the patient should be on bed rest. Assessing the device would be a next step in managing the patient's need, not the immediate intervention. Administering preordered pain medication may be appropriate, but the immediate intervention would be to elevate the head of the bed to relieve ICP. Neurology may need to be consulted, but the priority for this patient is to immediately relieve the pressure by elevating the head of the bed.

58. A) Cardiac tamponade
Cardiac tamponade's early symptoms are also late symptoms and include exertional dyspnea, chest pain, restlessness/agitation, tachycardia, and low blood pressure. ICP symptoms include headaches, nausea and vomiting, weakness, and papilledema. SVCS symptoms include swelling of the neck and face and distended veins. SCC symptoms include pain, weakness, and sensory loss.

59. B) Pulsus paradoxus
Pulsus paradoxus, a decrease in blood pressure of more than 10 mmHg with inspiration, is found in more than 75% of patients with cardiac tamponade. Papilledema is a symptom of increased intracranial pressure. Pericardial friction rub could be a symptom of cardiac tamponade, but it is not an ominous finding. Jugular vein distention can cause tachycardia but not a decrease in blood pressure.

60. C) Spinal cord compression

Spinal cord compression occurs because primary tumors of the spinal cord or tumor invasion of the vertebrae causes the spinal cord to collapse. Pneumonitis is an inflammation of the lining of the lung that can result from some cancer treatments, including radiation. Tumor lysis syndrome results from rapid destruction of cancer cells as a result of treatment. Superior vena cava syndrome can occur when a tumor compresses the superior vena cava.

61. C) Targeted therapy

Targeted therapy agents act on specific molecules in the cancer cell to prevent growth and division or to limit the cell's life span. Chemotherapy involves administration of chemical agents that kill cancer cells, and frequently healthy cells, around the malignancy. Radiation therapy involves delivery of concentrated doses of radiation to kill cancer cells or shrink tumors. Immunotherapeutic agents improve the ability of the patient's own immune system to attack cancer cells.

62. B) "Local anesthesia is preferred because anesthesia with intubation may cause hypotension and cardiac arrest."

Local anesthesia is preferred because intubation during full anesthesia may cause life-threatening hypotension and cardiac arrest. Since this is an emergent situation, it is likely the anesthesiologist will recommend having the procedure because there are methods of administering anesthesia in a safe manner. Anesthesia with intubation could cause hypotension and cardiac arrest. Pericardiocentesis is a temporary removal of pericardiac fluid that would not address cardiac tamponade.

63. B) Flushing

Maintaining a flushing routine is essential with vascular access devices. Dressing changes prevent infection at the site. Diphenhydramine is a medication that treats anaphylaxis reactions. Extravasation is an infiltration or leaking of intravenous antineoplastics into tissues surrounding the site.

64. A) Checkpoint inhibitors and chimeric antigen receptor therapy

Checkpoint inhibitors and chimeric antigen receptor therapy, as well as tumor infiltrating lymphocytes and oncolytic vaccine therapy, are classifications of immunotherapies. PARP and proteasome inhibitors, EGFR and HER2, and RTK and TKIs are targeted therapy small-molecule inhibitors.

65. A) Predict outcomes and monitor response

Companion diagnostics use companion assays to predict outcomes and monitor responses in patients receiving targeted therapy. Identifying patients is an area of companion diagnostics but is not done using companion assay. Determining scheduling, dosing, and discontinuation of treatment is also an area of companion diagnostics but is not determined by companion assay. Targeted therapies interfere with the molecules responsible for cell growth and proliferation.

66. B) Peripherally inserted central catheter

A peripherally inserted central catheter ends in the superior vena cava. Peripheral and midline catheters are not considered central venous lines as they are shorter catheters. Intrapleural catheters are placed in pleural spaces.

67. C) "Your medication, bevacizumab (Avastin), prevents your cancer cells from growing."

Targeted therapies act directly on specific molecules within cancer cells. Bevacizumab (Avastin) is a targeted therapy drug that prevents cancer cell growth by inhibiting vascular endothelial growth factor A. There are chemotherapy drugs that potentiate the effects of radiation, but targeted therapy medications do not act in this manner. Paclitaxel (Taxol) is a chemotherapy drug. Mesna (Mesnex) is a bladder protectant used in conjunction with the chemotherapy drug ifosfamide (Ifex).

68. B) Living

Biotherapies are made from living organisms. They interfere with, mimic, or help cell function signals. Augmented organisms are used in specific targeted therapies such as T cell therapy and are built from the patient's own immune system. Dead organisms are not used in biotherapies. Biosimilars are biologic medical products that mimic a different U.S. Food and Drug Administration–approved drug.

69. B) Tumor escape has allowed any tumor cells to progress

Tumor escape occurs when the tumor is not recognized by the immune system and therefore does not respond to therapies. Immunotherapy enhances the immune system and works to overcome tumor escape; therefore, it would not be the reason for progression of tumors. Cytokines failing to stimulate and regulate the immune system would not contribute to such aggressive metastasis. Monoclonal antibodies target tumor antigens that are harbored in certain people, but are not correlated with tumor escape or progression of tumor cells.

70. B) Educate patient on adverse events

Education about adverse events is very important in the biotherapy. Adverse side effects need to be treated right away so that therapy doses can be maintained. Hypoglycemia and hypertension are not side effects typically associated with biotherapy. Input and output education would not be needed as the patient would not need to monitor this.

71. C) Blood cells need to be reprogrammed with tumor antigen receptors

In CAR-T, T cells are harvested from blood, "reprogrammed" with tumor antigen receptors, and then infused into the patient. Although blood can be obtained from a donor for the procedure (allogenic), CAR-T is typically performed using the patient's blood (autologous). Red blood cells play no role in the therapy. The patient will need to be rehospitalized for infusions after cells have been augmented, so it cannot be completed in a single day.

72. C) Vaccinations

Cancer vaccinations condition the patient's immune system to generate its own response to tumor growth. In chimeric antigen receptor therapy, T cells from the patient's blood are modified to target cancer cells before being reinfused into the patient. Checkpoint inhibitors are agents that block checkpoint proteins, allowing T cells to remain active against cancer cells. Proteasome inhibitors refer to targeted therapy.

73. C) Targeted therapy

Targeted therapy interferes with specific molecules involved with tumor growth and progression. Chemotherapy's action is to destroy cancer cells. Immunotherapies use, stimulate, augment, or suppress cells of the patient's immune system. Radiation therapy kills tumor cells by damaging cell structures and preventing further growth of tumors.

74. B) Immunotherapy

Immunotherapies use, stimulate, augment, or suppress cells of the immune system. Targeted therapy interferes with specific molecules involved with tumor growth and progression. Chemotherapy and radiation therapy act directly on the cancer cells.

75. C) "Your port can be used for the high infusion pressure of CT contrast."
A power injectable implanted port can withstand the high infusion pressure of CT contrast. This device is used for chemotherapy infusions, scans, and lab draws to prevent the patient from getting temporary catheters placed at each appointment. The nurse can keep the port needle in place for the CT, and then remove it; it does not remain in place for the entire treatment duration. There is no reason to insert a peripheral catheter because the implantable port can be used for the CT contrast.

76. D) Target molecule
VEGF, or vascular endothelial growth factor, is a target molecule for one class of targeted therapy. Target molecules are classified by their role in cancer cell growth, migration, and metabolism. Chimeric antigen receptor T cells and checkpoint inhibitors are used in different types of immunotherapy.

77. D) Monitoring for fluid volume excess
The renal cancer patient is in danger of fluid volume excess and will have daily, not weekly, weights and vital signs. The nurse will encourage fluids, not limit them, unless they are contraindicated.

78. D) "I will need to complete an abdominal assessment."
Patients on opioids are susceptible to constipation, and the nurse will need to complete an abdominal assessment. One bowel movement a week is not appropriate for any patient, especially one taking opioids. It is not appropriate to assume that the patient is not constipated or to tell them they are fortunate not to have diarrhea.

79. D) Use an air or water mattress on the patient's bed
The patient with impaired integument will benefit from an air or water mattress to relieve pressure points. The family will turn the patient every 2 hours, complete a skin assessment every 4 hours, and refrain from massaging impaired areas due to risk of further injury.

80. A) "Sexual dysfunction is likely because of damage to the nerves."
In women, radical cystectomy involves removing the bladder, uterus, fallopian tubes, ovaries, anterior vaginal wall, and sometimes the urethra. Nerve damage and resulting sexual dysfunction are common. The patient will not be able to have children. It is inappropriate to suggest that sexual function will improve or that the patient's partner will find them less attractive.

81. B) Collect cultures from blood and other potential sites of infection

Neutropenia accompanied by fever strongly suggests infection. It is imperative to obtain cultures from all potential sites of infection, including blood, before initiating microbial therapy, as the microbiology and sensitivity panels play a crucial role in selecting appropriate antibiotics. Evaluation of potential drug–drug interactions, as well as patient comfort and family education, are important nursing roles, but they would not be next in the sequence of tasks.

82. B) The patient will use assistive devices when ambulating

The care plan will include use of assistive devices and repositioning of the patient every 2 hours, not 4 hours. The patient will not be capable of performing active range of motion on affected limbs. It is not necessary for the nurse to always ambulate the patient; other staff or family can assist.

83. B) Proto-oncogene

RAS is a proto-oncogene, a gene that regulates normal cell growth. It is not a tumor suppressor gene (one that inhibits uncontrolled growth), a caretaker gene (one that repairs genes), or a chromosome translocation (an instance of a piece of one chromosome moving to another chromosome).

84. B) Germline mutations

Alterations that occur in the *BRCA1* and *BRCA2* genes are among 853 known germline mutations that increase an individual's risk of developing cancer. Carcinogens are environmental factors that increase an individual's risk of developing cancer. Somatic mutations are noninherited mutations caused by carcinogens. *BRCA1* and *BRCA2* are examples of mutations that increase an individual's risk of developing breast cancer, not examples of breast cancer itself.

85. C) Angiogenesis

Angiogenesis is the creation of new blood vessels, which provides cancer cells access to nutrients and oxygen. Cell proliferation, or an increase in the number of new cells, is dependent on angiogenesis. Energy metabolism and oncogenetic division are not linked with blood vessel creation.

86. A) Point mutation

A point mutation occurs in one single DNA location or one single base pair. A germline mutation is an inherited mutation. Single switch is an on-off switch in processivity within the full genetic sequencing and is not a term used to describe this phenomenon. Genetic defects are a variety of different mutations in genes that may not be specific to the one specific location or strand of DNA.

87. B) Spleen

The spleen is a secondary lymphoid organ that helps to fight against antigens in the blood. The thymus is part of the primary lymphoid system and plays a role in the maturation of lymphocytes. The thyroid gland and liver are not considered lymphoid organs or tissues.

88. A) Metastasis

Metastasis occurs when cancer cells spread from the initial tumor site to distant organs in the body. Metastasis may sometimes be classified as stage IV disease. While stage III involves invasiveness to the surrounding tissue and lymph nodes, it does not involve full metastases to distant organs. Perineural invasion and extracapsular spread are mechanisms by which cancer cells begin to spread.

89. B) High-risk human papillomavirus (HPV)

The high-risk HPV vaccine is recommended by the American Cancer Society for the prevention of cervical cancer. The hepatitis B vaccine prevents hepatitis B, which may contribute to development of liver cancer. The shingles vaccine prevents herpes zoster virus infection, and the influenza vaccine prevents influenza; they are not associated with cervical cancer.

90. B) Chemical

Bile, tears, and perspiration are natural chemical barriers that are part of the innate immune system. Physical (e.g., mucous membranes) and cellular (e.g., cytokines) barriers are additional natural barriers in the innate immune system. Extrinsic barriers are not a classification of the innate immune system.

91. B) Wear clothing that covers the skin and a hat with a wide brim

The American Cancer Society recommends wearing clothing that covers as much skin as possible and a hat with a brim wide enough to shade the face, ears, and neck. According to the American Cancer Society, direct sun exposure should be avoided during the hours of 10 a.m. to 4 p.m., when UV rays are most intense. Tanning booths and sun lamps should be avoided altogether, and sunscreen with an SPF of 30 or higher should be used.

92. D) Hepatitis B virus (HBV)

HBV is known to be associated with liver cancer. *Helicobacter pylori* is a bacteria associated with some stomach cancers. HIV-1 is associated with Kaposi's sarcoma and B-cell lymphoma. EBV is associated with nasopharyngeal cancers, Burkitt and Hodgkin lymphomas, and stomach cancer.

93. D) "Most cancer survivors do return to work."

Most cancer survivors return to work. The Americans with Disabilities Act prohibits discrimination based on disability, including cancer. The Act requires that employers offer reasonable accommodations to allow cancer survivors to meet their job responsibilities. It would be inappropriate and nontherapeutic to dismiss the patient's concern by telling them not to worry or to seek other employment.

94. B) Secondary

Secondary prevention focuses on limiting the seriousness or impact of cancer through early detection. Screening of asymptomatic individuals is an example of secondary prevention. Methods of primary prevention, such as vaccination, are aimed at preventing disease by reducing risk factors or increasing resistance. Tertiary prevention applies effective therapies to decrease morbidity and mortality. Quaternary prevention is not a prevention level associated with oncology.

95. D) Palliative

Palliative measures emphasize comfort and reduce symptom burden. Preventive measures lessen the effects of expected disabilities. Restorative rehabilitation refers to the patient returning to the same level of functioning as before treatment. Supportive measures help provide patients with accommodations to deal with the effects of treatment.

96. A) 15 to 39 years

Cancer survivors in the 15 to 39 years age range are more likely to be uninsured or underinsured and need consistent follow-up. Individuals from birth to age 5 years are generally covered by the insurance of their parent or legal guardian, or they may qualify for alternative insurance coverage, such as state Medicaid plans. Individuals age 40 to 64 years generally have more financial stability to afford adequate healthcare coverage. Patients age 65 years and older qualify for Medicare and supplemental insurance.

97. A) Educating the patient about prosthetic bras

Supportive rehabilitation services assist patients with minimizing debilitating changes. For the patient with breast cancer, they would include educating a post-mastectomy patient about the availability of prosthetic bras. Ice therapy during treatment is preventive. A return to a previous level of function is considered restorative. Antiemetics during treatment are preventive and do not relate to rehabilitation after treatment.

98. B) Restorative

Restorative rehabilitation refers to the patient's returning to the same level of functioning as before treatment. Preventive rehabilitation lessens the effects of expected disabilities. Supportive help provides patients with accommodations to deal with the effects of treatment. Palliative measures emphasize comfort and reduce symptom burden.

99. C) Recurrence

The patient's young age; testing being conducted, such as blood work; and learning a friend has cancer are often triggers for the patient who fears recurrence. Fatigue might promote anxiety, but it is a less likely cause of this patient's concern. Rejection and treatment decisions are not relevant to what the patient is currently feeling.

100. C) Distress thermometer rating scale

One component of the National Comprehensive Cancer Network (NCCN) distress thermometer assesses emotional concerns that may be related to the fear of cancer recurrence. The American Society of Clinical Oncology CINV grading scale is an emetogenic potential scale used for chemotherapy. The National Cancer Institute's mucositis grading scale is for scoring the severity of oral mucositis. The American Cancer Society's pain diary helps patients keep a record of pain intensity and properties.

101. D) Safe sex information and possible late physical effects of treatment on reproductive systems

The American Cancer Society and Children's Oncology Group guidelines suggest that safe sex information and possible late physical effects of treatment on reproductive systems be discussed. Anatomy information is important, but it should not be discussed exclusive of other information. Discussion of abstinence is not a recommendation of the American Cancer Society and Children's Oncology Group; rather, information on safe sex is recommended. Whether sexual health content should be minimized so parents can discuss it with the patients themselves is a decision to be made prior to the counseling session.

102. D) Psychosocial

Psychosocial assessment includes social history, coping skills, anxiety, depression, fear of recurrence, and support systems. Prevention is related to past medical history. Physical and mobility are physical assessments.

103. C) To any patient diagnosed with cancer throughout the rest of their lifetime

Patients are considered cancer survivors at diagnosis and throughout the rest of their lifetime. The definition of cancer survivor includes anyone affected by the patient's diagnosis, including family members, caregivers, and significant others. The definition applies at diagnosis, not at initiation or conclusion of treatment, and it is not limited by length of survival or age at diagnosis.

104. B) A counselor to discuss sexual and social concerns and a primary provider/oncologist to assess physical issues

Sexual concerns involve physical, social, and emotional components that should be referred to specialists in those areas. The nurse should not delay referral. Referral to only a counselor or only a primary oncologist will not provide the full complement of professionals needed to address the patient's issues.

105. A) Nausea

Ondansetron (Zofran) is an antiemetic that may be used to treat nausea or vomiting. An antiemetic would not be an appropriate intervention for constipation, pain, or delirium.

106. A) POLST

An advance directive is a legal document that identifies a person's medical care wishes in the event they are not able to make their own decisions. A POLST (physician orders for life-sustaining treatment) is a directive specifically documenting instructions in the case of cardiopulmonary arrest. A power of attorney is an individual designated to make decisions on behalf of an incapacitated patient. A DNR is a do-not-resuscitate document stating the wishes of the patient to not be resuscitated based on the preferences in the advance directive.

107. C) Dyspepsia

Gastrointestinal upset, including dyspepsia, nausea, and ulcers, is one of the most common side effects of NSAIDs. Because neutropenia, rash, and headache are not typically caused by this class of drug, the nurse would not focus on them in their assessment of the patient.

108. B) Refer the patient for further evaluation and psychosocial services

A score of 4 or greater on the NCCN distress thermometer indicates a significant level of distress and warrants further evaluation and/or referral. Providing antidepressant medication is out of the nurse's scope of practice. Reevaluating the patient's score does not address the issue of the patient's distress. Documenting the score in the patient's chart should be done, but it is not the most appropriate next step.

109. C) Evaluating the need for each medication and working with the provider to simplify the regimen

Dysphagia is common in patients nearing the end of life. The most appropriate intervention for patients who are unable to swallow pills is to evaluate the need for each medication and simplify the regimen as much as possible. Some medications should not be crushed. Referral to speech therapy and education on medication adherence are not appropriate actions for this patient.

110. B) Lorazepam

Lorazepam is a benzodiazepine, the preferred class of drugs for seizure control in end-of-life care. While gabapentin and levetiracetam are antiepileptic medications, they are not the drugs of choice for end-of-life seizure management. Morphine is typically used for pain and respiratory distress rather than seizure management.

111. A) Patient's religious/spiritual background, beliefs, and preferred practices

The spiritual assessment should include identification of the patient's religious/spiritual background, preferences, beliefs, rituals, and preferred practices and should be incorporated into the nursing diagnoses and nursing plan of care. This helps the nurse to provide individualized patient-centered care and meet patient needs. The nurse should recognize their own religious/spiritual beliefs and not impose them on patients. A spiritual assessment is part of a holistic assessment of the patient. Socioeconomic status does not have a bearing on religious/spiritual assessments but can influence how the patient views cancer prevention or access to healthcare.

112. B) The patient's cultural and religious beliefs and norms

Cultural and religious beliefs and norms can lead to varied responses to advanced cancer and end-of-life discussions, so the nurse should understand what these mean to the patient. Hospice services can take place in the home, in an inpatient hospice center, or in a skilled nursing facility. Insurance information and clinical trials are not appropriate topics for this conversation.

113. C) Breasts may become enlarged from this type of therapy

Endocrine therapy for prostate cancer carries gynecomastia as a side effect. Libido is likely to decrease, and fertility can be affected. The medication is more likely to cause hair loss rather than hirsutism.

114. D) "Are there certain cultural or spiritual practices we can facilitate for you during your treatment?"

Diverse cultures have different norms and behaviors, which may have a major impact on all aspects of the cancer experience. The primary need of the patient is to address cultural and spiritual practices so the patient can feel more inclined to accept and be adherent in treatment. Simply asking how the patient feels about what the healthcare team can do to help does not directly address the primary need in the patient. Asking what cultural practices or herb and supplement regimens have been or are being engaged in is important but does not address the primary need of the patient receiving culturally appropriate care.

115. B) 45-year-old patient with terminal lung cancer

Oncology patients at greatest risk for sexual intimacy issues are adolescents, older adults, and those with a terminal illness. Therefore, a 45-year-old patient with terminal lung cancer is at the highest risk of experiencing these issues.

116. A) Reproductive medicine

A 27-year-old patient who was assigned female at birth should be referred to reproductive medicine prior to initiating chemotherapy to discuss fertility preservation options if the patient is considering having children in the future. Referral to psychiatry, pain management, and a free wig program may be indicated, but do not take priority, because fertility preservation is time-sensitive.

117. C) Lymphedema

Lymphedema is a late effect of certain surgeries or radiation that removes or damages lymph nodes, resulting in fluid accumulation. Lymphadenopathy is the enlargement of lymph nodes. Lymphoma is a type of hematologic malignancy. Endolymph is a type of fluid in the inner ear.

118. B) PLISSIT

PLISSIT (permission, limited information, specific suggestions, intensive therapy) is a discussion model that facilitates the discussion of intimacy between nurses and patients. CAGE assesses alcohol use, and ADPIE (assessment, diagnosis, planning, implementation, and evaluation) is an acronym for general provider care. Motivational interviewing is a discussion technique that elicits the patient's motivation to change behaviors.

119. C) Late effect
A late effect begins following the completion of treatment and can even occur years later. A long-term side effect starts during treatment and continues even after treatment ends. Acute side effects are typically sudden and short-term. Hypothyroidism is common after radiation to the neck, so this is likely a related effect.

120. D) Opioid use
Opioid use during treatment is one of the highest contributors to fatigue. Concurrent chemoradiation, rather than single-agent chemotherapy, is more likely to cause fatigue. Weight loss, rather than obesity, is more associated with fatigue. While smoking can contribute to fatigue as well, it is less impactful than opioid use.

121. D) Applying heat packs to the affected area
Elevation of the affected extremity, maintaining a healthy weight, and avoiding prolonged standing are evidence-based practices to decrease lymphedema. It is advised to avoid heat or cold because extreme temperatures can worsen lymphedema.

122. B) Young adults
Young adults have been found to have a higher risk of altered body image. Research shows that survivors of childhood cancers do not have an increased prevalence of altered body image compared with controls. While middle-aged and older adults may have altered body image, young adults tend to be at the highest risk.

123. B) "Hair loss will typically begin 2 weeks after you start chemotherapy; your hair will start to regrow 6 to 8 weeks after you receive your last dose."
The typical course of chemotherapy-induced alopecia begins 2 weeks after chemotherapy starts, and hair regrows 6 to 8 weeks after chemotherapy is completed. It does not occur within a day after starting chemotherapy, nor does regrowth begin immediately after completing treatment. Alopecia is typically not permanent, and it affects body hair as well as hair on the head.

124. B) Irritable bowel disease
Irritable bowel disease is a contraindication to having an orthoptic neobladder procedure because the new bladder is constructed from intestinal tissue. History of nephrolithiasis, recurrent urinary tract infections, and herpes simplex virus are not considered contraindications.

125. B) 68-year-old patient with renal insufficiency

Renal insufficiency and age older than 65 years both pose a greater risk for NSAID-related toxicities. History of cirrhosis, migraines, and breast cancer do not, in isolation, pose a problem for taking NSAIDs.

126. B) Single oral temperature of 101°F

The threshold for neutropenic fever is defined as a single oral temperature of 101°F or an oral temperature of 100.4°F sustained over 1 hour; this requires urgent intervention with antibiotic therapy. Rectal temperatures are typically not performed on neutropenic patients.

127. D) Opioid withdrawal

Opioid withdrawal occurs when opioid medication is stopped abruptly and includes symptoms such as nausea, diarrhea, perspiration, anxiety, and insomnia. Opioid withdrawal is not necessarily indicative of an addiction. While a panic attack can present with similar symptoms, the fact that the patient recently ran out of oxycodone should prompt increased concern for withdrawal. A medication allergy would typically not present 2 days after taking the medication.

128. B) It can take 2 to 4 weeks for the medication to start having an effect

Selective serotonin reuptake inhibitors (SSRIs) such as sertraline (Zoloft) can take 2 to 4 weeks to begin having a therapeutic effect, which is important for patients to understand. SSRIs should not be stopped abruptly. The medication is more likely to cause insomnia than somnolence. Although the medication may cause dizziness, the patient should be cautioned against driving only while dizziness may impair the activity; there is no clear contraindication to driving merely because sertraline is prescribed.

129. D) Meditation

Meditation is an example of a mind–body intervention that aims to help one's mind to improve the function of the body. Tai chi is an example of exercise therapy. Biofield therapy is a type of energy therapy. Chiropractic therapy is a manipulative, body-based method.

130. A) Exercise therapy

Tai chi is an example of exercise therapy. Manipulative therapy, mind–body intervention, and energy therapy are other forms of complementary and alternative medicine.

131. B) "While many herbal supplements are safe, we do not yet know how they interact with nivolumab."

It is still unclear how herbal supplements interact with programed cell death protein 1 (PD-1) and programmed death-ligand 1 (PDL1) inhibitors, and it is best to avoid these while on treatment until more data are obtained. It is inappropriate to declare that herbs are safe to take across the board because many interact with other drugs. It is also inappropriate to disregard the topic of herbal supplements or instruct the patient to take them on off-days only because this will not necessarily prevent interactions.

132. C) Natural products and mind–body practices

The NCCIH categorizes complementary health techniques into two subgroups: natural products (e.g., vitamins, herbs) and mind–body practices (e.g., massage, hypnotherapy). The NCCIH does not designate techniques by whether they are evidence-based, theoretical, approved, experimental, safe, or risky.

133. A) At initial cancer diagnosis

Palliative care should ideally begin at the initial diagnosis of advanced cancer to optimize symptom management throughout the course of the disease. It is not reserved for the progression of a disease or for when life expectancy is 6 months or less. Palliative care is not just for pain management; it addresses a broad scope of symptoms.

134. A) Complete blood count (CBC) with differential

Acupuncture may increase the risk of infection or bleeding in patients with neutropenia or severe thrombocytopenia; therefore, a CBC with differential should be reviewed if the patient plans to undergo acupuncture. BMP, liver enzymes, and thyroid panel would not be helpful in determining the potential safety of this therapy.

135. A) Bone marrow

The bone marrow is the primary site of hematopoiesis. A minority of hematopoiesis occurs in the liver and spleen, particularly in children. The lymph nodes transport immune cells but do not produce them.

136. D) "I will need to forgo all doctor visits to be eligible."

To qualify for Medicare-covered hospice care, a patient must have Medicare Part A, must consent to hospice care, and must have an estimated life expectancy of 6 months or less as documented by the referring physician and hospice director. Forgoing doctor visits is not a stipulation of hospice eligibility.

137. A) You may experience bone pain with this medication

The most common side effect of G-CSF is bone pain and arthralgia. While the G-CSF may prevent neutropenia, it is still important for patients to follow neutropenic precautions. Fever is not a typical side effect and would be more concerning for infection. G-CSF is generally given preemptively to prevent neutropenia.

138. C) 880/mm³

An ANC of 500/mm³ to 999/mm³ is considered a grade 3 neutropenia. An ANC of 1,600/mm³ or 1,800/mm³ is considered a grade 1 neutropenia. An ANC of 490/mm³ is considered a grade 4 neutropenia.

139. B) Radiation therapy kills tumor cells and minimizes damage to other organs

One of the main benefits of radiation therapy is its ability to kill tumor cells and halt their spread while minimizing damage to surrounding tissues and organs. Radiation therapy requires extensive pretreatment planning and is not always covered by insurance. It also requires a multidisciplinary team of physicians, nurses, physicists, and radiation therapists.

140. B) Check complete blood count (CBC) with differential

A patient who received carboplatin and docetaxel is at high risk for developing neutropenia, and the nadir typically occurs 7 to 14 days after infusion. Chills, malaise, and dysuria should raise suspicion of infection and prompt a CBC with differential to assess whether this patient is neutropenic. While a UA may also be warranted, determining whether the patient is neutropenic takes priority. Auscultating the patient's lungs and bowel sounds is part of a thorough physical exam but is not the most important next step.

141. C) To determine the radiation treatment and target volume

Simulation is done using imaging such as a CT scan to identify the target lesion and the volume of radiation to be used. While the patient should get oriented to the treatment process and will need to lie still, this is not the purpose of simulation. Simulation is not done for the purpose of assessing a tumor's sensitivity to radiation.

142. C) Mitosis

Ionizing radiation is optimally effective when cells are undergoing mitosis. It is not as effective during the growth and DNA synthesis phase. Rest is not part of the cell cycle.

143. A) Brachytherapy

Brachytherapy is a method of radiation in which the radiation is delivered within the tumor bed or very close to it. Intensity-modulated radiation therapy, stereotactic radiosurgery, and proton beam therapy are all types of external beam radiation.

144. A) 1 Gy = 100 rad

Rad and gray (Gy) are units of radiation dosing. 1 Gy is equal to 100 rad, and 1 rad is equal to 1 cGy.

145. A) "Radiation to the head and neck can cause delayed hypothyroidism."

Following radiation to the head and neck, patients should have their thyroid labs checked, as radiation can cause delayed hypothyroidism. While the radiation oncology team can order follow-up blood work, a patient's primary care provider will retain primary responsibility for ordering annual labs. Radiation does not necessarily increase a person's risk of hyperlipidemia. Blood work can identify and rule out cancer recurrence.

146. D) "Proton therapy will likely cause less damage to surrounding tissue."

The overall benefit of proton therapy in comparison to radiation therapy is that it is likely to cause less damage to tissue surrounding the tumor site. It is not necessarily a shorter course of treatment. It is a relatively newer modality and is not yet ubiquitous or used for many cancer types.

147. B) "Have you noticed brittle hair and nails or intolerance to cold?"

A patient with a history of radiation to the head and neck is at significant risk for hypothyroidism. Fatigue and weight gain are common symptoms of hypothyroidism, as are brittle hair and nails and intolerance to cold. Inquiring about dyspnea on exertion, rash, and depression would not be the most helpful questions in following up on this patient's symptoms.

148. A) Integumentary

Dermatologic toxicities are very common during radiation treatment and typically begin in the second week of treatment, with the potential to intensify quickly. Although it is important to thoroughly assess the entire patient, including their cardiovascular, digestive, and immune status, the priority for this patient would be a skin evaluation.

149. C) 125 to 129 mmol/L
The normal range for sodium is 135 to 145 mmol/L. A level of 130 to 134 mmol/L is considered mild hyponatremia. A level of 125 to 129 mmol/L is considered moderate hyponatremia. A level below 125 mmol/L would be considered severe hyponatremia.

150. B) Avoid nonsteroidal anti-inflammatory drugs (NSAIDs)
Patients with DIC should avoid NSAIDs, as these medications can increase bleeding risk. Avoiding fresh flowers is important for patients with neutropenia, which is not applicable to DIC patients. Patients should avoid strenuous activity. A low-fat, high-protein diet is not particularly beneficial for these patients.

151. A) Sputum and blood cultures should be obtained before starting the vancomycin
It is important to obtain cultures before starting antibiotics, as the antibiotics may affect the results. While it is important to start the vancomycin quickly, the cultures take precedence in order to identify the pathogen. Two sets of blood cultures are typically performed to minimize risk of contamination. Sputum should optimally be collected whether or not the patient reports dyspnea.

152. C) Gram-positive bacterial infections
Gram-positive bacterial infections are the most common cause of sepsis in the United States. Gram-negative bacterial infections are also a substantial cause but are not as common as gram-positive ones. Viral and fungal infections can also cause sepsis but are less common.

153. C) Providing patient education on esophageal and oral cancers
It is important to educate patients on the dangers of smokeless tobacco and its association with other cancer types, such as pancreatic, oral, and esophageal carcinomas. Chewing tobacco is not associated with lung cancer. Applauding the patient would not be appropriate. The patient is not eligible for lung cancer screening.

154. D) Placing the patient on oxygen
The patient's presentation is consistent with septic shock. The most immediate need is to address the patient's hypoxia by providing supplemental oxygen. An EKG and labs should be done but are not the most immediate need. Administering acetaminophen for fever is also not the priority at this time.

155. A) Cancer incidence is higher above age 55 years

The risk of developing cancer increases with age, with 87% of all cancer diagnoses occurring after age 55 years. Cancer does not peak between 30 and 50 years, nor is it highest in childhood and after age 60 years. Cancer does not affect all age groups equally.

156. A) Hispanic/Latinx patients

Hispanic/Latinx patients have the highest incidence of cervical cancer. African American patients have a lower incidence but the highest mortality rate for cervical cancer. White and Asian patients have lower incidence rates of cervical cancer.

157. A) Maintain good oral hygiene with regular dental visits

Xerostomia is a common long-term side effect among patients receiving radiation to the head and neck. These patients are at higher risk for developing dental cavities, and it is therefore important for them to maintain good oral hygiene. Acidic foods and hydrogen peroxide would likely be caustic. Fluoride toothpaste should be used, not avoided.

158. C) African American patients

African American patients are significantly more likely to die of prostate cancer than their White counterparts. Asian and Hispanic/Latinx patients are not at highest risk for developing prostate cancer but would still be screened.

159. B) Wear a compression sleeve on your right arm while flying

Patients who receive radiation to the breast are at increased risk for lymphedema on the treated side. Even if lymphedema has not manifested yet, compression sleeves should be worn while on an airplane because this can trigger the accumulation of fluid. Strenuous lifting should be avoided on the treated side, not the untreated side. There is no need to take prophylactic antibiotics or to avoid submerging the treated breast in water.

160. C) Auscultate the patient's lungs

A patient with dysphagia is at risk for aspiration pneumonia. As the patient presents with dyspnea and a productive cough, it is most important for the nurse to perform a lung exam to assess for signs of pneumonia. Guaifenesin will not address the root cause and could mask an infection. The patient would be referred to speech therapy, but this is not the first priority. The patient's swallowing would be properly assessed before recommending that the patient continue eating.

161. A) Ductal adenocarcinoma

Ductal carcinoma constitutes 70% to 80 % of breast cancer diagnoses. Lobular carcinoma makes up 10% to 15% of cases. Papillary and inflammatory carcinoma are much rarer forms of breast cancer.

162. A) Luminal A tumors

Luminal A tumors are typically low grade with high levels of estrogen receptor expression and respond well to endocrine therapy. Luminal B and normal-like breast tumors have similar prognoses that are worse than that for luminal A tumors. Basal tumors hold the worst prognosis and will not respond to endocrine therapy.

163. A) The tumor is well differentiated—the tumor cells look similar to those of the original tissue

The Bloom–Richardson scale is the most widely used system for histologic grading of breast cancer. Grade 1 indicates a well-differentiated, low-grade tumor. A poorly differentiated tumor would be classified as a grade 3. Bloom–Richardson grading does not provide information about whether the cancer has metastasized to lymph nodes or elsewhere.

164. B) Human papillomavirus (HPV)

The classification of an oropharyngeal cancer as HPV positive or negative helps with prognosis and treatment planning. EBV is associated with nasopharyngeal, rather than oropharyngeal, carcinomas. HER2 status is relevant in breast cancers and mutations in the EGFR gene are relevant in lung cancers.

165. C) Tumor, nodes, metastases

TNM is the main staging system for cancer and helps to determine prognosis and appropriate treatment. It describes the size of the tumor (T) and whether the cancer has spread to lymph nodes (N) or metastasized to other parts of the body (M). Neither type of tumor nor genetic mutations are described by this system. While the French system includes mitotic count and tumor necrosis, those concepts are not a part of the TNM staging system.